FOURTH EDITION

CONCEPT MAPPING

A CRITICAL THINKING APPROACH

TO CARE PLANNING

Pamela McHugh Schuster, PhD, RN, FNP-BC
Professor of Nursing
Youngstown State University
Youngstown, Ohio

F.A. Davis Company • Philadelphia

F. A. Davis Company
1915 Arch Street
Philadelphia, PA 19103
www.fadavis.com

Printed in the United States of America

Last digit indicates print number: 10 9 8 7 6 5 4 3 2 1

Aquisitions Editor, Nursing: Megan Klim
Content Development Manager: Darlene D. Pedersen, RN, MSN
Content Project Manager II: Amy Romano
Illustration and Design Manager: Carolyn O'Brien
Electronic Project Manager: Tyler Baber

As new scientific information becomes available through basic and clinical research, recommended treatments and drug therapies undergo changes. The author(s) and publisher have done everything possible to make this book accurate, up to date, and in accord with accepted standards at the time of publication. The author(s), editors, and publisher are not responsible for errors or omissions or for consequences from application of the book, and make no warranty, expressed or implied, in regard to the contents of the book. Any practice described in this book should be applied by the reader in accordance with professional standards of care used in regard to the unique circumstances that may apply in each situation. The reader is advised always to check product information (package inserts) for changes and new information regarding dose and contraindications before administering any drug. Caution is especially urged when using new or infrequently ordered drugs.

Library of Congress Cataloging-in-Publication Data

Schuster, Pamela McHugh, 1953- , author.
  Concept mapping : a critical-thinking approach to care planning / Pamela McHugh Schuster. -- Fourth edition.
    p. ; cm.
  Includes bibliographical references and index.
  ISBN 978-0-8036-3848-8
  I. Title.
  [DNLM: 1. Patient Care Planning. 2. Audiovisual Aids. 3. Concept Formation. 4. Nursing Process--organization & administration. WY 100.1]
  RT42
  610.73--dc23
                    2015017961

This book is dedicated to nursing students and clinical faculty who use concept care maps to form clear mental models of patient situations and deliver excellent patient care.

This book is also dedicated to my husband, Fred, and to my children, Luke, Leeanna, Patty, Isaac, Brent, and Maggie, and grandchildren Adam, Lucas, Julianna and Cameron.

PREFACE

The purpose of this book is to teach nursing students how to use concept mapping theory to develop a concept care map, which is to be used in the direct care of patients and to communicate with members of the health-care team. Concept mapping is a diagrammatic teaching and learning strategy that allows students and faculty to visualize interrelationships between medical diagnoses, nursing diagnoses, assessment data, and treatments. Concept care maps result in a clear mental model of the patient health state and situation. Students must learn to share relevant information with the specific aim of creating a shared mental model with members of the health-care team to prevent errors that result in patient injuries and death.

The fourth edition of patient care maps is updated and revised based on continued use of concept care maps in varied clinical settings and the recommendations of the faculty and students who have been working with concept care maps since the first publication. This edition includes both basic and complex patient case studies, and integrates the 2010 ANA Standards of Nursing Practice and updated NANDA Nursing Diagnoses. The online resources include 14 additional case studies so that students can practice creating maps for various clinical settings as they advance through a nursing program, a Test Yourself Quiz to assist students in determining that they understand the theory behind creating a care map, and podcasts explaining the history and theory of concept mapping, as well as detailing the individual steps for creating a concept map.

The concept care map comprises a five-step process. Before developing a care map, the student must perform a patient assessment. From the assessment data, the student develops a skeleton diagram of the patient's health problems (step 1). The student then analyzes and categorizes specific patient assessment data (step 2) and indicates relationships between nursing and medical diagnoses (step 3). In step 4, the student develops patient goals, outcomes, and nursing strategies for each nursing diagnosis. Step 5 is to evaluate the actual patient response to each nursing strategy and to summarize clinical impressions. Care mapping enables the student to recognize the relationships between medical and nursing care problems, including integration of pathology, medications, treatments, laboratory and diagnostic testing. Using this care map process, the student:

- Identifies the primary patient care problems using specific evidenced-based assessments,
- Analyzes patient profile data and categorizes data to describe problems, and documents each problem within a box on the care map,
- Draws lines between boxes to indicate relationships.
- Assigns numbers to the problems to indicate their priority,
- Develops a goal, outcomes, and strategies for each problem,
- Uses care maps to select appropriate strategies to provide effective care,
- Uses care maps as the basis for documentation in patient medical records, and
- Uses care maps to participate in developing a shared mental model of the patient's health status and situation with members of the health-care team to prevent patient harmful events.

After the theoretical discussion of each step to develop the care map, the book presents case studies and end of chapter exercises that the student can use to gradually develop the ability to clinically reason and formulate accurate and complete nursing diagnoses and then develop the individualized plan of care. Concept care maps promote clinical reasoning and development of an accurate mental model of the patient situation. My best wishes for much success in nursing, and I hope you find this book a useful guide for designing excellent plans of patient care.

A Note about Usage

To avoid both sexism and the constant repetition of "he or she," "his or her," and so forth, masculine and feminine pronouns are used alternately throughout the text.

CONTRIBUTOR LIST

Louise A. Aurilio, PhD, RN-BC,
  NE-BC, CNE
Professor Emeritus of Nursing
Youngstown State University
Youngstown, Ohio
C-section with Gestational Diabetes
  (OB)
Newborn with Jaundice (OB)

Kelly Clark, MSN, RN
Clinical Instructor of Nursing
Youngstown State University
Youngstown, Ohio
Bipolar with Psychosis (P)

Susan Lisko, DNP, RN, CNE
Associate Professor of Nursing
Youngstown State University
Youngstown, Ohio
Appendectomy (MS)

Mary Beth Lukach, MSN, RN, CNS
Associate Lecturer of Nursing
Kent State University Trumbull
Warren, Ohio
Depression with Polysubstance
  Abuse (P)

Valerie O'Dell, DNP, RN, CNE
Associate Professor of Nursing and MSN
  Program Director
Youngstown State University
Youngstown, Ohio
Newborn with Jaundice (OB)
Newborn of Mother with Gestational
  Diabetes (OB)
Vaginal Delivery with Laceration and
  Repair (OB)
Vaginal Delivery for Gravida 9 (OB)

Jill E. Rankin, DNP, RN
Assistant Professor of Nursing
Youngstown State University
Youngstown, Ohio
Osteosarcoma with Chemotherapy
  (Peds)
Sickle Cell Crisis (Peds)

Sueann Rendano, MSN, RN
Instructor of Nursing
Youngstown State University
Youngstown, Ohio
Vaginal Delivery with Laceration
  and Repair (OB)
Vaginal Delivery for Gravida 9 (OB)

Molly Roche, MSN, CNS, RNC
Instructor of Nursing and RN-BSN
  Coordinator
Youngstown State University
Youngstown, Ohio
Parkinson's Disease and Trauma Due
  to Falling (MS)

Kimberly A. Serroka, DNP, RN
Professor of Nursing
Youngstown State University
Youngstown, Ohio
Cystic Fibrosis in Hospital (Peds)
Respiratory Syncytial Virus (Peds)

Cynthia M. Shields, MSN, ACNP-BC,
  CCRN
Assistant Professor of Nursing
Youngstown State University
Youngstown, Ohio
Opioid Overdose with Renal Failure
  and Respiratory Depression (CC)
Sleep Apnea with Respiratory
  Failure (CC)

Mary Shortreed, MSN, RN, CNE
Instructor of Nursing
Youngstown State University
Youngstown, Ohio
Osteoarthritis and Dementia (LTC)

Bonnie L. Thompson, MSN, RN
Instructor of Nursing
Youngstown State University
Youngstown, Ohio
Orthostatic Hypotension, COPD (MS)
Arthroplasty of Right Hip,
    Osteoarthritis (MS)

Nancy H. Wagner, DNP, RN, CNE
Associate Professor of Nursing and
    Chairperson
Youngstown State University
Youngstown, Ohio
Cystic Fibrosis (Peds)
Respiratory Syncytial Virus (Peds)
Tonsillectomy (Peds)

Amy Weaver, PhD, RN, CNE
Assistant Professor of Nursing
Youngstown State University
Youngstown, Ohio
Hip Fracture with Delayed Wound
    Healing, Osteoporosis (LTC)

(LTC) *Medical-Surgical - Long Term*
    Care Adult
(MS) *Medical-Surgical - Hospitalized*
    Adult
(P) *Psych*
(CC) *Critical Care*
(OB) *OB - Hospitalized Mother-*
    Newborn
(Peds) *Pediatrics - Hospitalized*
    Children

REVIEWERS

Billi Blake, MSN, BSN, Ed.D., CNE
Associate Dean of Nursing, Director
   of BSN Program
St. Johns River State College
Orange Park, Florida

Connie Booth, MSN, RN
Nursing Program Chair/Instructor
Des Moines Area Community College
Boone, Iowa

Kim Ewertz, MS, BSN, CTE
Faculty- Nursing
Morgan Community College
Fort Morgan, Colorado

Nancy Hall, DNP, RN
Associate Professor, Nursing
Bemidji State University
Bemidji, Minnesota

Bonita Kershaw, MSN, RN, CHSE RN
Nursing Instructor/Learning Resource
   Center Coordinator
St. Joseph School of Nursing
Nashua, New Hampshire

Mary T. McGill, CCNS, Clinical Nurse
   Specialist
Nursing Faculty- Instructor
Radford University
Radford, Virginia

Rebecca Presswood, MS, RN
Nursing Instructor
Blinn College
Bryan, Texas

Joyce Stanley, MSN/CNS, RN
Assistant Professor
Learning Enhancement Center
   Coordinator
The University of North Carolina
   at Pembroke
Pembroke, North Carolina

Karen Ursel, PhD, MHA, BSN
Senior Nursing Instructor
University of New Brunswick
Moncton, New Brunswick
Canada

Tammy Willis, MS
Nursing Faculty
Metropolitan Community College
Kansas City, Missouri

CONTENTS

'TWAS THE NIGHT BEFORE CLINICAL . . .

'Twas the night before clinical, and all through the house not a creature was stirring . . . except for you! There you are, with books piled high around you, trying to get ready to give safe and competent nursing care to the patients you have been assigned in the morning. It is late, and you are tired. What if there was a way for all the information you have gathered on your patients to just "come together", make perfect sense, and form a simple, complete care plan? If you have ever found yourself in this situation, this book is for you. It was written to help you quickly and efficiently organize and analyze patient data and develop a working care plan that is referred to as a concept "care" map. A concept "care" map is the plan used to give daily nursing care to a patient. The concept care maps you develop will be practical and realistic; they will be implemented and evaluated during the clinical day. And best of all, there is very little writing to do! No more tedious writing of nursing care plans.

The purpose of this book is to teach you how to develop a concept care map, which is to be carried in your pocket on the clinical area and used in the direct care you provide your patient and in communication with members of the health-care team. In addition, it is very important for you to understand how your performance and your concept care map will be evaluated by your clinical faculty.

The purpose of this chapter is to describe the theoretical basis for concept care maps and to provide an overview of what they are, how they are developed, and how they are used during patient care. In addition, the chapter introduces general standards for guiding and evaluating patient care within managed care systems. Managed care principles are used in almost all health-care delivery systems. The purpose of managed care is to decrease costs while maintaining the quality of health-care services. The implications of managed care are far-reaching, and they guide the development of nursing care plans. Later chapters will lead you step by step through each aspect of developing and using concept care maps.

What Are Concept Care Maps?

Concept care mapping is an innovative approach to planning and organizing nursing care. In essence, a concept care map is a diagram of patient problems and nursing strategies to eliminate those problems. Your ideas about patient problems and treatments are the "concepts" that will be diagrammed. In this book, the term *concept* means idea. Developing clinical concept care maps will enhance your critical thinking skills and clinical reasoning, because you will visualize priorities and identify relationships in clinical patient data clearly and succinctly. Concept care maps result in a clear mental model of the patient's health state and situation. Students must learn to share relevant information with the specific aim of creating a shared mental model with members of the health-care team to prevent errors that result in patient injuries and death.[1] In 2000 the Institute of Medicine[2] first reported 48,000 to 98,000 deaths per year due to errors—an average of one death every 5 to 10 minutes—spawning the patient safety movement in health-care delivery over the past decade. The concept care map is a strategy that can be used to delineate what needs to be communicated among caregivers about the patient's health state and situation.[3]

Concept care maps are used to:

▶ Organize patient data
▶ Analyze relationships in the data
▶ Establish priorities
▶ Build on previous knowledge
▶ Identify what you do not understand
▶ Enable you to take a holistic view of the patient's situation[4]
▶ Participate in developing a shared mental model of the patient's health status and situation with members of the health-care team to prevent harmful events[3]

The templates for the concept care map are located in Figures 1.1, 1.2, and 1.3.[4] Take a few minutes to study them. You will be using these templates to outline patient problems; organize patient data on abnormal results of physical and psychosocial assessment, treatments, medications, and laboratory results; develop goals and outcomes; and list what you will be doing to address each problem. Figure 1.1 is the "sloppy copy," where you will be writing down short notations about a patient's problems by grouping data under problem areas. It does not have to be perfect; it takes time to think critically about how to categorize data correctly under problems, and sometimes you may change your mind about where data fit into the clinical picture you are developing about your patient. The "final edition" in Figure 1.2 is the care plan you submit after the clinical day is over, after you have had more time to critically evaluate what happened during your clinical experiences with the patient. Bring your sloppy copy and the goals, outcomes, and nursing strategies in Figure 1.3 to the clinical agency.

The Theoretical Basis of Care Mapping

Concept care maps have roots in the fields of education and psychology.[5,6] Concept maps have also been called cognitive maps, mind maps, and meta-cognitive tools for teaching and learning.[7,8]

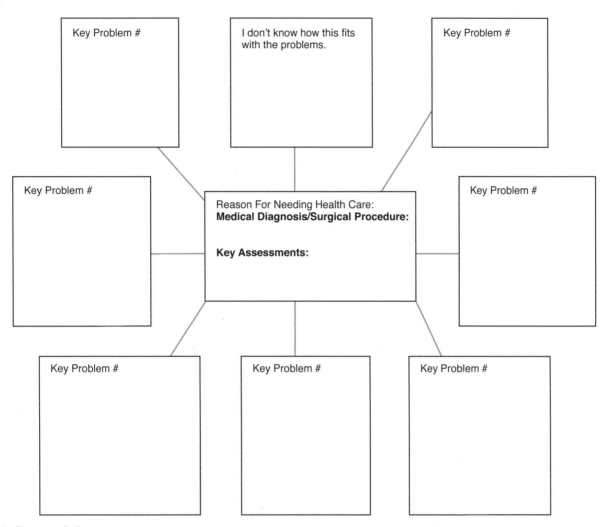

● Figure 1.1   Sloppy copy pre-conference. Carry this in your pocket at all times!

They have been used in many classroom settings as teaching tools to get important ideas to stick in the minds of students. Nursing educators have recognized the usefulness of this teaching and learning strategy in summarizing and visualizing important concepts, and there is a growing body of knowledge on this topic.[9-13]

From the field of education, Novak and Gowin[5] developed the theory of meaningful learning and have written about "learning how to learn." They have theoretically defined concept maps as "schematic devices for representing a set of concept meanings embedded in a framework of propositions." They further explain concept maps as hierarchical graphical organizers that serve to demonstrate the understanding of relationships among concepts. This theoretical definition and explanation is highly abstract; simply stated, concept maps are diagrams of important ideas that are linked together. The important ideas you need to link are patient problems, abnormal physical and psychosocial assessment data, medications, laboratory results, and treatments for the patient's problems. The concept maps you will be developing are for patients in clinical settings, so they are named concept "care" maps. You will use this special concept "care" map to guide your nursing care of patients, and during communications with all members of the health-care team to develop a shared mental model of the patient situation.

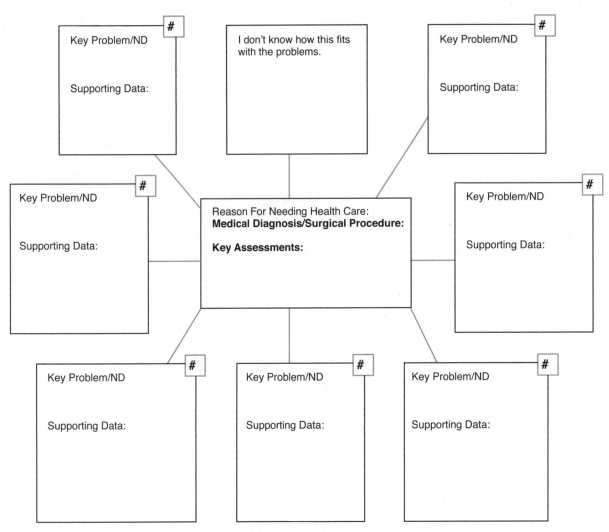

● Figure 1.2   Final edition. Give this to your clinical instructor the day after clinical.

The educational psychologist David Ausubel[6] has also contributed to the theoretical basis of concept mapping through the development of assimilation theory. Concept maps help those who write them to assimilate knowledge. The premise of this theory is that new knowledge is built on preexisting knowledge, and new concepts are integrated by identifying relationships with those concepts already understood. Simply stated, we build and integrate new knowledge into what we already know. By diagramming, you build the structure about the relationships between important concepts related to the care of your patient. Concept maps help to identify and integrate what you already know and help reveal what you do not understand. This means that although you have ideas about patient problems or treatments, you may not be sure of how those problems and treatments should be integrated into a comprehensive plan. Once you recognize what you do not understand and can formulate questions, you can seek out information. Concept care maps help identify what you know and what you need to learn to provide quality patient care. The concept care map you create will evolve as you continue to assess and intervene with your patient. You will be adding to the concept care map throughout the clinical day, and using it to communicate with your clinical faculty and other members of the health-care team.

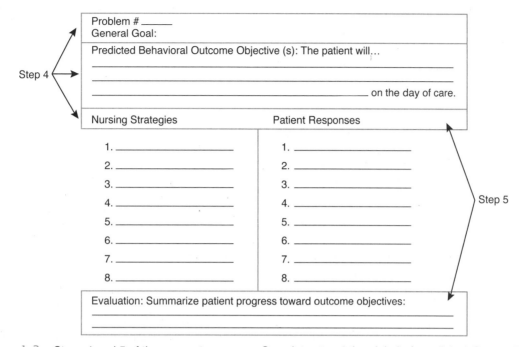

Step 4

Problem # _____
General Goal:

Predicted Behavioral Outcome Objective (s): The patient will...
_____
_____
_____ on the day of care.

Nursing Strategies	Patient Responses
1. _____	1. _____
2. _____	2. _____
3. _____	3. _____
4. _____	4. _____
5. _____	5. _____
6. _____	6. _____
7. _____	7. _____
8. _____	8. _____

Step 5

Evaluation: Summarize patient progress toward outcome objectives:
_____
_____

● Figure 1.3 Steps 4 and 5 of the concept care map. Complete step 4 the night before clinical. Step 5: Evaluation of patient responses. Complete step 5 the day of clinical.

Concept Care Mapping and Critical Thinking Yield Clinical Planning

Concept care mapping requires critical thinking. A widely accepted view of critical thinking by many nurse educators was developed by the American Philosophical Association: "Critical thinking is the process of purposeful, self-regulatory judgment. This process gives reasoned consideration to evidence, contexts, conceptualization, methods, and criteria."[14] In developing a clinical concept care map, critical thinking is used to analyze relationships in clinical data. Thus, critical thinking used in developing concept care maps builds clinical reasoning skills. Critical thinking and clinical reasoning are used to formulate clinical judgments and decisions about nursing care. In 2000, the National League for Nursing Accrediting Commission's *Report on Planning for Ongoing Systematic Evaluation and Assessment of Outcomes* defined critical thinking specific to the discipline of nursing as "The deliberative _non-linear_ process of collecting, interpreting, analyzing, drawing conclusions about, presenting, and evaluating information that is both factually and belief based."[15] In the 2010 edition of

Nursing: Scope and Standards of Practice, the American Nurses Association (ANA) explains that the "nursing process in practice is not linear as often conceptualized. . . . Rather, it relies heavily on the bi-directional feedback loops from each component"[16(p3)] Concept care maps are nonlinear and will be used to collect, interpret, analyze, draw conclusions about, present, and evaluate patient information, and to communicate with members of the health-care team.

Although concept maps have been used in a number of different ways in various disciplines, including nursing, the focus of this book is on developing concept "care" maps for the purposes of clinical nursing care planning. You need to organize the concept "care" map prior to the care of the patient, which will help you organize and prioritize what needs to be done to promote optimal patient outcomes for the clinical day of care. The important ideas that must be linked together are the medical and nursing diagnoses, along with all pertinent clinical data, including the subjective and objective physical and emotional problems and the underlying pathology, medications, laboratory data, and treatments. Concept care maps can be used to promote critical thinking and clinical reasoning about patient problems and treatment of problems. Through concept care mapping of diagnoses and clinical data, you can evaluate what you know about the care of a patient and what further information you need to provide safe and effective nursing care.[17]

Take, for instance, a situation where a certain drug or treatment may not make any sense to you as you analyze the entire clinical picture. It is very important to ask questions of your clinical faculty about what does not seem to fit the clinical picture, because the questions you ask can result in avoiding medication or treatment errors. In the past, there have been times when patients have needed changes in their medications or treatments based on the findings of nursing students. So never hesitate to ask questions of your faculty and other members of the health-care team. This is so important, in fact, that a special place has been provided on the care map template, labeled "I don't know how this fits with the clinical problems." Place any information that you do not understand in this box. Perhaps there are drugs you cannot find in your references the night before clinical, or you may wonder why a patient needs a particular drug or treatment. The visual concept care map diagram of relationships among diagnoses allows you, your clinical faculty, and members of the health-care team to exchange views on why relationships exist among the problems and treatments and to construct a shared mental model of the patient's health state and situation. It also allows you, your faculty, and other members of the health-care team to recognize the need for further assessment and questioning, to avoid medication or treatment errors.

Overview of Steps in Concept Care Mapping

The nursing process is the foundation of the concept care map or any other type of nursing care plan. The nursing process involves assessing, diagnosing, planning, implementing, and evaluating nursing care. These steps of the nursing process are related to the development of concept care maps and the use of care plans during patient care in clinical settings. Subsequent chapters will give the details of care mapping with learning activities, but it is important for you to have an initial overview.

Preparation for Concept Care Mapping

Before developing a concept care map, the first thing you must do is gather clinical data. This step corresponds to the assessment phase of the nursing process. You must review patient records to determine current health problems, medical histories and chronic illness, abnormal physical and psychosocial assessment data, medications, and treatments. This assessment must be complete and accurate, because it forms the basis for the concept care map. You may have the opportunity to meet a patient briefly the day before you begin care. In just 5 minutes of interacting with a patient—even by simply introducing yourself and watching the patient's response—you can gain a wealth of information about the patient's mood, level of comfort, and ability to communicate. Chapter 2 will focus on how to gather clinical data.

Step 1: **Develop a Basic Skeleton Diagram**

Based on the clinical data you collect, you begin a care map by developing a basic skeleton diagram of the reasons your patient needs health care. The initial diagram is composed of your clinical impressions after you have reviewed all the data initially collected on a patient. In the first case study, the patient is admitted to the nursing home long term care facility because he has Alzheimer's disease and can no longer take care of himself at home. As shown in Figure 1.4a, the reason for seeking care is in the middle of the template, in the box labeled "Reason for needing health care." The health care this refers to may include the reason for hospitalization, extended care, or a visit to the outpatient center. Sometimes the focus of a visit may be on high-level wellness; for example when a patient is seen for a screening examination and the aim is to maintain wellness and prevent problems.

Then, around this reason for seeking care, arrange the clinical problems that were determined based on the initial patient assessments—these problems are associated with the reason for seeking health care. In this case study,

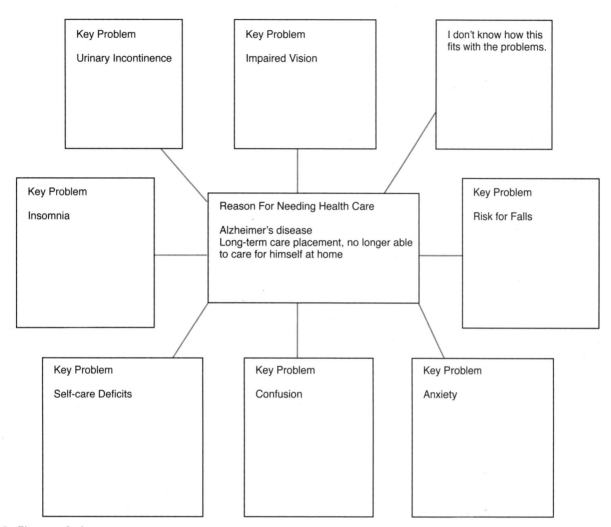

● Figure 1.4a   **Step 1:** Write the key problems the patient has, based on the data collected. The key problems are also known as the *concepts*. Start by centering the reason for seeking health care (often a medical diagnosis). Next, list the major problems you have identified based on the assessment data collected on the patient.

the problems identified include confusion, self-care deficits, urinary incontinence, risk for falls, impaired vision, insomnia, and anxiety. The general statements of patient problems will eventually be written as nursing diagnoses.

The American Nurses Association (ANA) Social Policy Statement[16] indicates that the focus of nursing practice is on the diagnosis and treatment of human responses to health states. The concept care map diagram reflects the ANA practice policy statement because the human responses are located around the health state of the patient. Nursing care will be focused on the human responses.

The concept care map diagram is primarily composed of nursing diagnoses resulting from the health state, flowing outward from the central figure like spokes on a wheel. The concept care map diagram focuses strictly on real nursing care problems based on collected data; it does not focus on potential problems. At this stage of care planning, it is most important to recognize major problem areas. You do not have to state the nursing diagnosis yet. Write down your general impressions of the patient after your initial review of data.

Labeling the correct diagnosis is difficult for many students. At this point, it is more important to recognize major problem areas than to worry about the correct nursing diagnostic label. If you recognize that the patient is confused, write that down. You are first looking for the big picture. Later, you can look up the correct nursing diagnostic label and decide if the diagnosis should be *Chronic Confusion or Impaired Memory.* Initially, just write, in whatever words come to mind, what you think are the patient's problems. Recognizing that something is wrong with the patient is more important than applying the correct label. Chapter 3 will expand on step 1 on formulating basic diagrams of problems.

Step 2: *Analyze and Categorize Data*

In this step, you must analyze and categorize data gathered from the patient's medical records and your brief encounter with the patient. By categorizing the data, you provide evidence to support the medical diagnoses and nursing problems/ diagnoses. You must identify and group the most important assessment data related to the patient's reason for seeking health care. The data you are collecting will depend on your level in the nursing program and the patient population. In this first example, you are in your first semester in nursing, learning fundamentals, and are providing care to a patient in a nursing home.

In Figure 1.4b, study the nursing problems/ diagnoses flowing outward from the patient's reason for seeking health care. Listed under each problem/nursing diagnosis is the clinical evidence that led you to conclude that the problem or diagnosis was appropriate to this patient with Alzheimer's disease.

When making a concept care map, you must write important clinical assessment data; that may include pathophysiology, treatments, laboratory values, medications, and medical history data related to each patient problem/diagnosis. The assessment data collected depends on your course level in the nursing program. As you advance, you will be sifting through and sorting out the often voluminous amount of data that is available on a patient. The sicker the patient, the more complex the analysis. You need to list assessment data regarding physical and emotional indicators of problems or symptoms of pathology under the appropriate problem/diagnosis. For example, physical indicators of problems from the data on the

Alzheimer's disease patient include "oriented to name only," "thinks his father is still alive," and "thinks he is currently a construction worker building the dining room in the nursing home." These are listed under the problem of *Confusion.* Emotional indicators of problems are "apprehension about daily activities" and "feeling lost when his wife is not present." These are listed under the nursing diagnosis *Anxiety.* Depending on your course level, you must also list current information on diagnostic test data, treatments, and medications under the appropriate problems. For this case study, you are in fundamentals and have not yet taken pharmacology; you have a limited knowledge of diagnostic testing and medications, so these are not included on this concept care map.

When beginning to use concept care maps with medical and nursing diagnoses that are new to you, you may not always know how to categorize abnormal assessment findings. If you do not know where such information should go, list it in the "I don't know how this fits the problem" box of the template and ask for clarification from your clinical faculty. (This box is located in the upper right corner of Figure 1.4b.) At least you recognized that the patient data was important, even if you do not yet have the experience to see where it fits in the overall clinical picture of patient care. After discussion with the clinical faculty, you become aware that the data of history of hypertension and venous insufficiency, cold fingers, pale nail beds, and pacemaker, along with edema of the extremity, indicate a nursing diagnosis of *Ineffective Peripheral Tissue Perfusion*—beyond the level of your current fundamentals course—and that you should check further in a care plan book for details.

Sometimes you may think that symptoms apply to more than one nursing diagnosis, and they often do. You recognize that the patient is confused, but that observation could go under *Risk for Falls* or *Self-Care Deficits,* and is also a separate problem. It makes sense to place this symptom in more than one area. Therefore, you can repeat a symptom in different categories if it is relevant to more than one category.

Finally, you must determine the priority assessments that still need to be performed regarding the primary reason for seeking care; write them in the box at the center of the map

Figure 1.4b Step 2: Support problems with clinical patient **data,** including abnormal physical assessment findings, medical history, and emotional state. Also, identify **key assessments** that are related to the reason for seeking health care and put these in the central box. If you do not know what box to put data in, then put it off to the side of the map.

under "Key assessment" in Figure 1.4b. In deciding what the key assessments are, consider what the most important assessments would be if you were responsible for assessing a group of six to eight patients, as you one day will be as a nurse. These key assessments are your priority and must be done on first contact with the patient and carefully monitored throughout the clinical day. Focus on the key areas of assessment that must be performed to ensure that the patient's outcomes on the day of care are as expected. For the patient with Alzheimer's

disease, you would assess his neurological status and the safety of his environment. This step in the concept care mapping process appears in detail in Chapter 3.

Step 3: **Label and Analyze Relationships Among Nursing Diagnoses**

Next, you need to label nursing diagnoses and analyze the relationships among them, as shown in Figure 1.4c. You need to determine the correct diagnosis for the problem of confusion that may be

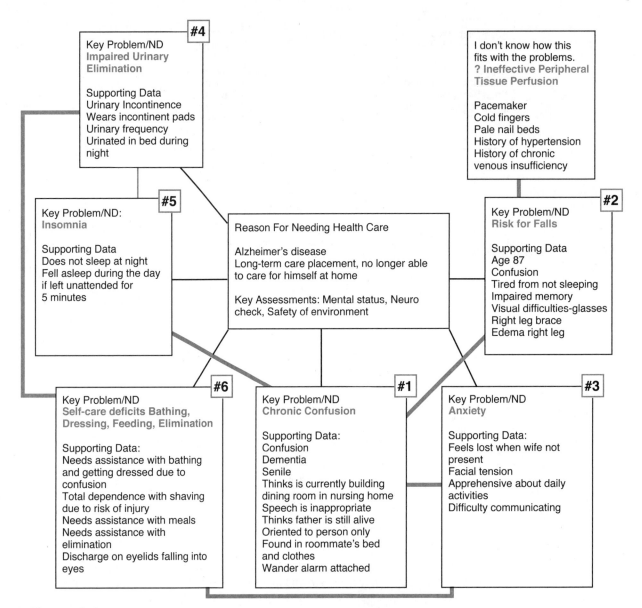

● Figure 1.4c   Step 3: Draw lines between related problems. Use numbers to prioritize problems. Lastly, label the problem with a **nursing diagnosis.**

labeled *Chronic Confusion or Impaired Memory.* After looking up definitions of these diagnoses, you conclude that *Chronic Confusion* is the most appropriate diagnosis.

You will need to prioritize your nursing diagnoses by numbering them. Your priorities are going to be what you think are the most important problems. All the problems you have identified are important, but attempt to number them.

Priorities do change throughout the clinical day; you may do your sloppy copy thinking that *Chronic Confusion* is going to be a top priority, but it may turn out that for your patient *Anxiety* is the major problem of the day. Therefore, use your sloppy copy to guess at the order of priority, but then use your final edition to accurately prioritize your diagnoses based on what happened during the clinical day.

You will also be drawing lines between nursing diagnoses to indicate relationships, as shown in Figure 1.4c. In this example, **Chronic Confusion** is related to **Risk for Falls, Anxiety,** and **Insomnia.** Be prepared to explain to your clinical faculty why you have made these links. Your faculty may want you to add the words that describe the relationship linkages. For example, why **Insomnia** and **Chronic Confusion?** In this case, the explanation is that the patient who is not sleeping will have decreased ability to function and increased confusion, and that will contribute to the state of disorientation. You will soon recognize that all the problems the patient is having are interrelated. You and your clinical faculty can see the whole picture of what is happening with the patient by looking at the map. Thus, concept care maps are a holistic approach to patient care. These issues will be expanded upon in Chapter 3.

Step 4: *Identify Goals, Outcomes, and Nursing Strategies*

On the template in Figure 1.4d you will write patient goals and outcomes and then list nursing strategies to attain the outcomes for each of the numbered diagnoses on your concept care map. General goals and behavioral outcome objectives are at the top of the template, with nursing strategies listed in the first column.

You will carry the sloppy copy of the care map, goals, outcomes, and strategy lists in your pocket as you work with the patient, and you will either check off nursing strategies as you complete them or make revisions in the diagram and strategies as you interact with the patient. The concept care maps with strategies are used during the implementation phase of the nursing process.

The nursing strategies include key areas of assessment and monitoring as well as communication strategies needed to establish effective nurse-patient relationships or collaborate with other members of the health-care team. To decrease paperwork, rationales for nursing strategies are not written down. Come prepared to verbally explain the rationales for your identified nursing strategies if you are asked by your clinical faculty. It is of course a professional responsibility to know why you are using each strategy, even though you are not writing it down.

Be prepared to review nursing strategies during the clinical preconference. Nursing strategies include what you are supposed to be carefully monitoring and includes a list of all appropriate treatments, medications, and patient teaching, depending on your level in the nursing program. Step 4, on goals, outcomes, and nursing strategies, will be expanded on in Chapter 4.

Step 5: *Evaluate the Patient's Responses*

This step is the written evaluation of the patient's physical and psychosocial responses. It is shown in the second column of Figure 1.4d. As you perform a nursing strategy, write the patient's responses. For example, you say in step 4, under the nursing diagnosis **Chronic Confusion,** that you will assess the patient's neurological status. In step 5, you will record orientation to person, place, time, and circumstances data across from your assessment of neurological status. Step 5 also involves writing your clinical impressions and inferences regarding the patient's progress toward expected outcomes and the effectiveness of your strategies to bring about these outcomes. This is an evaluation statement written to summarize progress toward the outcome objectives for each nursing diagnosis, found at the bottom of the template in Figure 1.4d. Step 5, on evaluation of outcomes, will be expanded on in Chapters 5 and 6.

As you progress in the nursing program, you will be required to build upon your knowledge of patient care and integrate knowledge of medications and laboratory data into the concept care map. The purpose of the following case study is to illustrate an acutely ill hospitalized patient and demonstrate how concept care maps may be used to simplify and summarize data for a more complex patient.

Complex Patient Step 1

In step 1 of concept care mapping, you develop a skeleton diagram with the reason for needing health care in the central box of the diagram and the patient problems fanning out around

Problem #_____ 1 _____ : Chronic Confusion
General Goal: Patient remains safe from harm in protected environment

Predicted Behavioral Outcome Objective (s): The patient will . . . be free of injury, wear wander guard, follow simple directions, remain calm on the day of care.

Nursing Strategies	Patient Responses (Evaluation)
1. Neuro Assessment	1. Alert & oriented to person only, PERRLA Follows simple directions
2. Make sure alarm attached to leg, alarm on exit door Hygiene products locked	2. Alarms remained intact, toxic substances locked in top bedside drawer
3. Give single simple instructions	3. Followed instructions
4. Speak in quiet tones	4. Seemed more relaxed & less frustrated
5. Use consistency & repetition	5. Understood most of conversation & all instructions
6. Use distraction	6. Easily distracted by change in conversation when became frustrated due to confusion
7. Make sure glasses are clean	7. Wore glasses all day except when getting shaved
8. Orient to place & time	8. Listened attentively while explained the time of day (morning), season (winter), and showed him which side of room was his

Summarize patient progress toward outcomes objectives: Patient remained free of injury, wore the wander guard, was able to follow simple directions, and remained calm. Need to continue assessment of neurological functioning and orient to place and time. Improvement in understanding directions and remaining calm by using communication strategies.

Problem #_____ 2 _____ : Risk for Falls
General Goal: Patient does not fall

Predicted Behavioral Outcome Objective (s): The patient will . . . remain free from falling on day of care.

Nursing Strategies	Patient Responses (Evaluation)
1. Assess risk for falls	1. Patient at risk due to age, confusion, insomnia, edema, & leg brace
2. Assist with ambulation Wear brace	2. Ambulated to PT and lunch Wears brace all day
3. Make sure glasses are clean & in place	3. Wore glasses all day except while shaving
4. Keep one side rail up	4. Side rail remained up
5. Dangle before standing	5. Always sat up with feet on ground before rising to a standing position
6. Use wheelchair if weak or tired	6. Did not have to use wheelchair, ambulated safely
7. Room clear of hazards	7. Room with obstructing furniture, no small items on floor
8. Shoes, slippers socks, nonskid	8. Nonskid shoes worn

Summarize patient progress toward outcomes objectives: The patient ambulated safely and remained free of falls, protective environment was maintained.

● Figure 1.4d   Step 4: Identification of goals, outcomes, and strategies. Step 5: Evaluation of patient responses.

that reason like spokes on a wheel. The skeleton diagram of a concept care map diagram for a complex patient is shown in Figure 1.5. In this case study example, the reason the patient was admitted to the health-care setting was for an abdominal abscess with bowel obstruction and for surgery. His problems include pain, skin integrity, elimination, cardiac output, mobility,

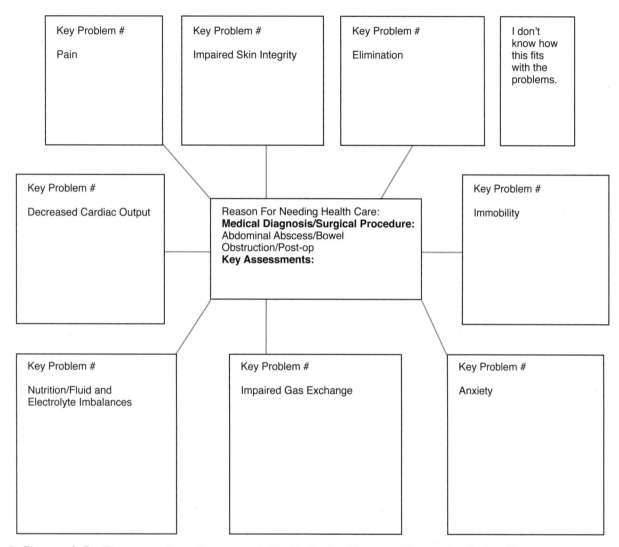

● Figure 1.5   The reason the patient was admitted to the health-care setting, and patient problems.

nutrition and fluid and electrolyte balance, gas exchange, and anxiety.

Complex Patient Step 2

In step 2, you analyze and categorize specific patient assessment data. Figure 1.6 shows the skeleton diagram of the reason for admission and resulting patient problems with assessment data to support each problem listed in the box under each problem. In this case study, physical and psychosocial assessment data, chronic illnesses, diagnostic test results, treatments, and medications are listed under the appropriate problems.

For example, physical indicators of problems from the data include labored respirations at a rate of 22 per minute, fatigue, and decreased breath sounds. These are listed under the patient problem of *Impaired Gas Exchange.* Emotional indicators of problems include the patient crying and verbalizing that he is nervous and saying that he knows he is going to die. These are listed under the patient problem of *Anxiety.*

You must think critically to place diagnostic test data, treatments, and medications under the appropriate category. For example, diagnostic tests include blood studies of white blood cells,

Key Problem
Pain
Abdominal abscess-
surgical wound
Mouth ulcers
Ca of bone/lung with
chronic pain
Demerol (meperidine)
Morphine

Key Problem
Impaired Skin Integrity
T = 100.5°F
Infection-Abscess-wound
2 drains, purulent drainage
Fecal material in drain
WBC = 12.9

Key Problem
Elimination
Foley
Check urine output >60 cc/h
Enlarged prostate
Proscar (finasteride)
Creatinine = 5
BUN = 22

I don't
know how
this fits
with the
problems.

Key Problem
Decreased Cardiac Output
Atrial fibrillation
Vitals = q4h
Rate = 128 (irregular)
BP = 113/60
K = 3.3
Lanoxin (digoxin)
PT = 17.5
PTT = 40.2
Fatigue

Reason For Needing Health Care:
Medical Diagnosis/Surgical Procedure:
Abdominal Abscess/Bowel
Obstruction/Post-op
Key Assessments:
Pain, Distention, Bowel Sounds,
I&O, Drainage & Wound

Key Problem
Impaired physical mobility
Ca of bone (history)
Chemotherapy (history)
Fall protocol
Lethargic/fatigued
Tubes (tripping)
Plexipulses

Key Problem
**Nutrition/Fluid and
Electrolyte Imbalances**
NPO
Mouth ulcers
NG tube
TPN
IV
139 lb, 5' 10"
Nystatin (mycostatin)
FBS = 147 (history of diabetes)
Dry skin
Anemic
Weakness

Key Problem
Impaired Gas Exchange
Ca of lung (history)
Radiation/chemotherapy (history)
Respiratory treatments
Decreased breath sounds rt lung
Incentive spirometry
Respirations labored, check q4h
RT = q4h, Ventalin (albuterol)
RR = 22
Oxygen = 5L
Hgb = 10
Fatigued

Key Problem
Anxiety
Surgery
Says he knows he's going
to die
Clenches his fists when he
can't do something
Chronic pain
Fidgets with his hands
Cries
Verbalizes he is nervous

● Figure 1.6   The reason the patient was admitted to the health-care setting, and patient problems, with assessment data added to support the final edition.

hemoglobin, and potassium. In this case, the white blood cells are listed with *Impaired Skin Integrity* and the abscessed wound, the hemoglobin with *Impaired Gas Exchange,* and the potassium with *Decreased Cardiac Output.* Oxygen and respiratory treatments are categorized with *Impaired Gas Exchange.* The medication morphine is categorized with **Pain**, albuterol (Ventolin) is categorized with *Impaired Gas Exchange*, and digoxin (Lanoxin) is categorized with *Decreased Cardiac Output.*

The medical history information is also listed under the patient problems. All chronic illnesses must be integrated on the care map. In this example, the patient has a history of chronic illness related to bone and lung cancer, atrial fibrillation, and an enlarged prostate. The bone and lung cancer chronic illnesses are listed under the nursing diagnoses of *Pain*, *Impaired Gas Exchange,* and *Impaired Physical Mobility;* atrial fibrillation is under *Decreased Cardiac Output,* and the enlarged prostate is listed under *Elimination.*

In step 2, you identify what you do not know by asking for clarification in the "I don't know how this fits the problem" box of the template, located in the right corner of the diagram. In this example, note that the reason for the medication Demerol is in question.

Symptoms often apply to more than one nursing diagnosis. The patient is lethargic and fatigued, but that observation could go under **Decreased Cardiac Output**, **Impaired Physical Mobility,** or **Impaired Gas Exchange.** A symptom may be placed in different categories under patient problems if it is relevant to more than one category.

Step 2 also involves determining the priority assessments that need to be performed regarding the primary reason for seeking care; these are written in the box at the center of the map under "Key assessment," as shown in Figure 1.6. For this patient, key assessments include pain, bowel sounds, abdominal distention, intake and output, the wound and drainage from it.

Complex Patient Step 3

In step 3, you label patient problems as nursing diagnoses, prioritize them, and indicate relationships between them, as shown in Figure 1.7. For example, it is important to distinguish whether respiratory and breathing problems should be labeled **Impaired Gas Exchange** or **Ineffective Airway Clearance.**

Next you prioritize problems/diagnoses by numbering them, in this situation the problems have been prioritized from 1 to 8. Priorities do change throughout the clinical day, you may do the sloppy copy thinking that **Pain** is going to be a top priority, but it turns out that your patient does not have any, and for him **Anxiety** is the major problem of the day. Therefore, use your sloppy copy to guess at the order of priority, but then use your final edition to accurately prioritize what happened during the clinical day.

Lines are drawn between nursing diagnoses to indicate relationships as shown in Figure 1.7. In this example, **Pain** is related to **Anxiety, Impaired Physical Mobility, Impaired Skin Integrity,** and **Imbalanced Nutrition.** Be prepared to explain to your clinical faculty why you have made these links. You may explain by writing the critical thinking that led you to conclude that the diagnoses were related. For example, why are pain and nutrition related?

In this case, the explanation is that the patient has mouth ulcers and an uncomfortable nasogastric tube, contributing to pain.

Complex Patient Steps 4 and 5

Steps 4 and 5 of this case study are shown in Figure 1.8. In step 4, you develop patient goals and outcomes and nursing strategies for each nursing diagnosis. Goals and outcomes are listed, followed by the listing of nursing strategies that include what needs to be assessed in addition to treatments and medications. Patient teaching should be listed under nursing strategies as appropriate for each problem. For example, patient teaching may involve slow, deep breathing and guided imagery under the nursing diagnosis **Anxiety.**

In step 4 it is important to list in the nursing strategy column when the nurse assigned to oversee the patient's care will be doing a treatment that you have not yet learned how to do. For example, under **Imbalanced Nutrition,** you may write that the patient needs total parenteral nutrition and care of the nasogastric tube but that these strategies will be done by the staff nurse since you have not yet learned how to provide them. By writing the treatments in the appropriate column, you demonstrate that you have recognized these nutrition-related treatments and their importance to the total care needed by the patient. Be prepared to discuss the basic purpose of the nursing strategies, even those you do not perform yourself.

In step 5, you evaluate the patient's response to each specific nursing strategy and summarize your clinical impressions. This step is the written evaluation of the patient's physical and psychosocial responses, shown in the second column in Figure 1.8. For example, you say in step 4, under the nursing diagnosis **Impaired Skin Integrity,** that you will monitor the patient's temperature. In step 5, you record those temperatures across from the nursing strategy. Step 5 also involves writing your clinical impressions and inferences regarding the patient's progress toward expected outcomes and the effectiveness of your strategies to bring about these outcomes. The box to write evaluation statements in to summarize progress toward the outcome objectives for each nursing diagnosis is found after the nursing strategy and patient response lists for each nursing diagnosis.

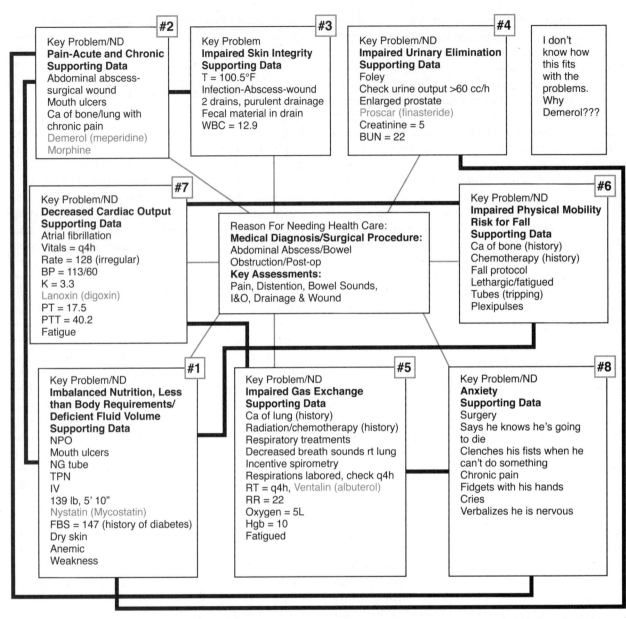

● Figure 1.7   Final edition with formulation of diagnoses, linkages between diagnoses, and prioritization of problems.

During Clinical Care: Keep It in Your Pocket

Throughout the clinical day, you and your clinical faculty will have an ongoing discussion regarding changes in patient assessment data, effectiveness of nursing strategies, and patient responses to those strategies. Keep the concept care map in your pocket; this way, everything that must be done and evaluated is listed succinctly and kept within easy reach. As the plan is revised throughout the day, take notes on the

● Figure 1.8
Steps 4 and 5 of the concept care map. Complete step 4 the night before clinical. Step 5: Evaluation of patient responses. Complete the day of clinical.

Step 4

Problem #_____5_____: Impaired Gas Exchange
General Goal: Maintain oxygenation

Predicted Behavioral Outcome Objective (s): The patient will...cooperate with RT, use oxygen, and breathing remains non-labored...on the day of care.

Nursing Strategies	Patient Responses
1. Assess breath sounds	1. Crackes throughout lung fields especially rt. base
2. Assess VS, especially respirations	2. 8:00 156/80 112-20; 12:00 126/58 88-20 (temp. above)
3. Maintain oxygen administration	3. Oxygen on at 5L continuous
4. Monitor hemoglobin	4. No new labs
5. Do CDB with respiratory therapy (RT)	5. RT did CDB after treatments
6. Perform incentive spirometry q2h	6. Pt. performed IS q2h

Step 5

Evaluation: Summarize patient progress toward outcome objectives: Breathing non-labored but crackes present, cooperative with treatments, elevations in pulse and BP may be due to pain as above.

Step 4

Problem #_____6_____: Impaired Physical Mobility/Risk for Falls
General Goal: Moves without injury

Predicted Behavioral Outcome Objective (s): The patient will...perform ROM, get up to the chair, and not fall...on the day of care.

Nursing Strategies	Patient Responses
1. Assess fatigue and strength prior to movement	1. Weak and tired
2. Safe environment (Fall protocol)	2. Personal items in reach
3. Side rails, low bed, call bell in reach	3. At all times
4. Compression devices used in bed	4. On while in bed
5. Perform ROM q2h	5. Done with bath & q2h
6. Get up in chair at bedside	6. Got up for 1h then became fatigued

Step 5

Evaluation: Summarize patient progress toward outcome objectives: Got up for an hour but is weak and tired. Performed ROM. High risk for falls due to weakness and fatigue.

Step 4

Problem #_____7_____: Decreased Cardiac Output
General Goal: Maintain cardiac output

Predicted Behavioral Outcome Objective (s): The patient will...have pulse and BP remain stable and electrolytes WNL...on the day of care.

Nursing Strategies	Patient Responses
1. Check VS q4h, especially BP & P	1. As above
2. Apical check with Lanoxin	2. 10:00 112
3. Assess circulation in extremities	3. Radials and pedals 3+ bilaterally
4. Listen for arrhythmias	4. Atrial fibrillation
5. Monitor	5. K=3.8

Step 5

Evaluation: Summarize patient progress toward outcome objectives: CV system stable.

Step 4

Problem #_____8_____: Anxiety
General Goal: Decrease anxiety

Predicted Behavioral Outcome Objective (s): The patient will...verbalize concerns...on the day of care.

Nursing Strategies	Patient Responses
1. Therapeutic communication, especially empathy, distraction, active listening	1. Verbalizes concerns about dying
2. Guided imagery	2. States it helps him relax
3. Teach slow deep breathing	3. Appeared more relaxed, less gimacing
4. Comfort touch	4. Held my hand when talking

Step 5

Evaluation: Summarize patient progress toward outcome objectives: Patient responded to anxiety interventions by verbalizing concerns.

● Figure 1.8
Continued

concept care map diagram, add or delete nursing strategies, and write patient responses as you go along. As your clinical faculty makes rounds and checks in on you and your patients, they can also refer to the concept care maps with goals, outcomes, and strategy lists you have developed as the basis for guiding your patient care.

Documentation

The concept care maps with strategies and patient responses will become the basis of your documentation. You will be using the revised plans and outcome evaluations as guides to make sure you have adequately documented patient problems, strategies, and your evaluation of patient responses. Documentation involves correctly identifying patient assessment data to record a problem, determining what to record about the strategies to correct the problem, and describing the patient's responses to the strategies. Assessment, strategies, and responses are all present in the concept care map. Concept care maps as the basis of documentation will be described in more detail in Chapter 7.

Medication Administration

Your concept care map will also be useful as you prepare to administer medications. By organizing the drugs to be administered under the correct problems, you demonstrate your knowledge of the relationship of the drug to the problems. You can also see the interactive effects of the drug related to the total clinical picture. For example, as you discuss digitalis (Lanoxin) administration under *Decreased Cardiac Output,* you and your clinical faculty can also see that the patient's potassium level is low. What is the relationship between low levels of potassium and digoxin administration? The answer is an increased risk of a toxic reaction by the patient to digitalis. Be prepared for your clinical faculty to ask you for the current value of potassium from the morning blood draw. Low potassium levels have to be corrected; in the meantime,

you can be assessing the patient carefully for adverse reactions to the drug. You can more easily integrate medications with laboratory values and pathology if the information is all neatly categorized under *Decreased Cardiac Output.*

In addition, you should write down scheduled times of medication administration next to the drugs. You may also highlight drugs on the map. Writing down administration times and highlighting drugs helps to organize information and remind you of the importance of the medication administration times. It also decreases the chance of medication errors.

Nursing Standards Of Care

Concept care maps are individualized plans of care built on critical analysis of patient assessment data, identification of medical and nursing diagnoses, determination of nursing strategies to be implemented, and evaluation of patient/healthcare consumers outcomes. Development, implementation, and evaluation of safe and effective nursing care are contingent upon nurses' knowing and following accepted standards of care. As you plan care for a patient, a primary question you must address is: What are the standards of care pertinent to my patient and specific to the applicable medical and nursing diagnoses? Nursing students often wonder, "Have I included everything necessary in this care plan? Am I doing everything I should be doing? Am I missing something?" Following standards of care ensures that you are doing everything possible to provide appropriate care to the patient. These standards may stem from several organizing agencies or principles.

Standards of the American Nurses Association

By law, nurses must follow guidelines for the safe and effective practice of nursing. These legal guidelines are called *standards of professional nursing practice.* The ANA has developed general standards of nursing practice, shown in Box 1-1. Concept care maps are in compliance with these general standards of care.

Box 1.1	AMERICAN NURSES ASSOCIATION STANDARDS OF PROFESSIONAL NURSING PRACTICE

1. The registered nurse collects comprehensive data pertinent to the health-care consumer's health and/or the situation.
2. The registered nurse analyzes the assessment data to determine the diagnoses or the issues.
3. The registered nurse identifies expected outcomes for a plan individualized to the health-care consumer or the situation.
4. The registered nurse develops a plan that prescribes strategies and alternatives to attain expected outcomes.
5. The registered nurse implements the identified plan.
   5A. The registered nurse coordinates care delivery.

5B. The registered nurse employs strategies to promote health and a safe environment.
5C. The graduate-level prepared specialty nurse or advanced practice registered nurse provides consultation to influence the identified plan, enhance the abilities of others, and effect change.
5D. The advanced practice registered nurse uses prescriptive authority, procedures, referrals, treatments, and therapies in accordance with state and federal laws and regulations.
6. The registered nurse evaluates progress toward attainment of outcomes.

Source: © By American Nurses Association. Reprinted with permission. All rights reserved.

Standards for Accreditation of Health-Care Organizations

Since July 2010, laws were enacted that placed accrediting agencies under the jurisdiction of the Centers for Medicare and Medicaid Services (CMS).[18] CMS makes decisions to grant deeming authority to accrediting organizations and determines the term. One example of an accrediting organization with deeming authority is the Joint Commission. The Joint Commission will only accredit hospitals that have written policies and procedures for nursing care. You must follow these specific policies and procedures for any nursing care you administer in order for the health-care agency to maintain its accreditation. Representatives of The Joint Commission travel the country and review these policies and procedures. If they are not current, The Joint Commission requires that they be updated if the agency desires to maintain its certification as an accredited health-care agency.

Fortunately for you as a student, fundamentals and medical-surgical textbooks provide general descriptions of procedures that are similar to what is required by your clinical agency. Your clinical faculty will inform you of any specific requirements of the clinical agency in which you are placed, either by explaining those requirements verbally or by referring you to the agency's procedure manual.

Standardized Nursing Care Plans

Many organizations have developed standardized nursing care plans for specific medical diagnoses. These standardized nursing care plans are based on typical nursing diagnoses of patients with particular medical problems. Many facilities have general nursing care plans for nursing care of patients that are commonly seen. For example, an orthopedic unit probably has a standardized care plan for the patient with a fractured hip, and the urology unit probably has a standardized care plan for the patient undergoing a transurethral resection of the prostate gland. In addition, hundreds of standardized care plans have been written and published, and many have been computerized for easy accessibility.

Therefore, while you are gathering data from a patient's records to prepare your care map, you also need to find out whether the agency has any standardized care plans available for you to use. If these plans are not available on the unit to which you are assigned, you can use published books of standardized care plans to make sure you have not missed any important aspects of care.

Health-Care Literacy and Patient Education Standards

All patients have the right to know what is wrong with them and how to manage their own care. Health literacy is the aim of patient education. Nurses play a key role in educating patients and ensuring that health-care literacy is attained. Most agencies have patient education materials available that are specific to various types of problems. You need to collect these materials when you collect information from patient records. As with standardized care plans, standardized teaching materials, such as booklets and movies, have been published that may be available for you and the patient as references. Teaching materials are usually geared toward a fifth-grade reading level. Materials given to patients must be carefully screened for content that is appropriate for the patients' individual needs and ability to comprehend the materials. Detailed information about integrating teaching materials with care maps appears in later chapters.

Insurance Company and Government Care Standards

The high cost of health care has led to a concerted effort by the government (which pays for Medicare and Medicaid) and health-care insurance companies to control costs. At the same time that costs are being controlled, the quality of health care is supposed to be ensured through careful management by health-care providers. The government and insurance companies have developed specific criteria for which services will and will not be reimbursed, depending on diagnoses. All medications, treatments, surgeries, and rehabilitation programs (literally everything done by health-care providers) has to be provided and documented according to government and

insurance company criteria for care, or the bills will not be paid. When bills are not paid by the government or insurance companies, health-care providers may never receive payment for services provided. In some cases, patients may be left with the bill. In that situation, patients may decide to go without needed health-care services because they cannot afford them.

Insurance companies and the government pay predetermined amounts of money to agencies or physicians providing care to patients. For example, if a patient has knee replacement surgery, the providers will receive a fixed amount of money for that service. Case managers, typically advanced practice nurses, are hired by insurance companies and health-care agencies to evaluate the types of care given to inpatients and outpatients, to monitor patient progress, and to coordinate the care of patients to guide their recovery while minimizing costs. These case managers are also known as resource managers, because they coordinate all services available to the patient. They must be aware of all resources available so they can make the appropriate linkages between patients and needed health care services.

Teams of health-care providers including physicians, nurses, pharmacists, dietitians, physical therapists, and social workers have developed standards that guide the treatment of patients. Instead of separate plans of care from the physician, dietitian, and others, the trend is for health-care providers to collaborate and develop one unified plan of care. This multidisciplinary plan is commonly called a *clinical pathway* or a *critical pathway*. There is careful sequencing of clinical patient care strategies over a specific period of time that all parties involved in the care of the patient agree to follow. Clinical pathways outline assessments, treatments, procedures, diet, activities, patient education, and discharge planning activities. Although clinical pathways are becoming a popular method of collaborative care planning, they are unfortunately not available for every diagnosis. Clinical pathways also vary slightly among clinical agencies.

As you prepare for a clinical care assignment, it is important that you know about the clinical pathway your patient is supposed to be following based on the patient's health condition. Because nurses often spend more time with patients than other health-care providers, nurses' clinical roles include communicating between caregivers to make sure that the patient is making steady progress in the expected direction toward the health goals enumerated on the clinical pathway. The nursing care plan and assessment is focused on identifying complications and quickly intervening to get the patient back on the clinical pathway, to resume rapid progress toward health goals.

Currently, a battle is raging between health-care providers and those who pay the bills for services, namely the government (for Medicare and Medicaid) and the insurance companies. At one time, physicians ordered whichever tests they felt necessary to diagnose problems and whichever treatments they deemed necessary to fix those problems. If a physician felt that a patient would benefit from an extra day in the hospital, the patient stayed in the hospital. If a physician ordered certain medications to treat the patient's problem, the patient received them. Now, physicians have been forced to use criteria established by insurance companies and the government for diagnosing, treating, admitting, and discharging patients—or the bill is not paid. In essence, the view of the insurance company and government is that physicians are free to treat patients as they deem necessary. However, if physicians deviate from the established standards and criteria for treatment, they are not paid. A few years ago, the standard used by those paying the bills was that patients were required to leave the hospital 24 hours after vaginal childbirth. The outcry from the public and from health-care providers grew so loud that the length of stay for vaginal delivery has now increased to 48 hours.

Although this is a simple explanation of the current state of affairs regarding payment for services and maintaining quality of care, it is a very complex problem. The complexity exists because the government and insurance companies differ on the types of payment plans and criteria that form the standards of care. In addition, the criteria are under constant revision.

Utilization Review Standards

Documentation of detailed assessments, accuracy of diagnoses, and appropriateness of treatments and follow-up are constantly reviewed in all health-care settings (such as private physicians' offices, outpatient facilities, and hospitals). Everything and everyone is under *utilization review*—the process of evaluating the care given by nurses, physicians, and all other health-care providers and agencies. It is nurses, primarily, who manage utilization reviews, armed with specific criteria for auditing individual health-care providers and the delivery of services in each health-care setting. These nurses are hired by health-care agencies and by insurance companies. Utilization reviewers do not usually have direct contact with patients; they review charts only. They judge the necessity and appropriateness of care and the efficiency with which care is delivered.

Managed Care in Hospital Settings

There is a direct relationship between the care standards described above and the management of care. Currently, nearly all patients who enter hospitals find themselves in managed-care delivery systems. Typically, patients entering health-care facilities have nurse case managers assigned to monitor and coordinate their progress through the health-care system. These case managers are experienced nurses, most of them holding advanced degrees or specialty certifications. These nurses manage hospital resources carefully and coordinate discharge planning. With strict criteria imposed by government and insurance companies to ensure rapid discharge from acute care facilities, all nurses must carefully document and justify complications and additional problems with patients to ensure that quality care is rendered and financial obligations are met (that is, the bills are paid by the government and insurance companies). These nurses monitor patient progress and especially track high-risk patients, as well as all patients with complications. These hospital-based nurse case managers interact with service providers and insurance providers; thus, they are considered resource managers. It is essential to make links for patients to home health services, transitional care units, long-term care facilities, and other agencies to provide quality care.

CHAPTER 1 SUMMARY

The purposes of concept care maps include assisting you with critical thinking, analyzing clinical data, planning comprehensive nursing care for your patients, and providing the basis for communication with members of the health-care team to create a shared mental model to prevent patient harm. A concept care map is based on theories of learning and educational psychology, and is a diagrammatic teaching/learning strategy that provides you with the opportunity to visualize interrelationships between medical and nursing diagnoses, assessment data, and treatments. The visual diagram of problems and the list of anticipated outcomes and strategies are personal pocket guides to patient care, and they form the basis for discussion of nursing care between you and your clinical faculty.

Before developing a concept care map, you must perform a comprehensive patient assessment. Then, in step 1 of concept care mapping, you develop a skeleton diagram of health problems. In step 2, you analyze and categorize specific patient assessment data. In step 3, you label diagnoses, prioritize them, and indicate relationships between nursing and medical diagnoses. In step 4, you develop patient goals, outcomes, and nursing strategies for each nursing diagnosis. In step 5, you evaluate the patient's response to each specific nursing strategy and summarize your clinical impressions.

The development of concept care maps is based on understanding and integrating accepted standards of patient care. Standards of care are derived from the nursing practice standards of the ANA and The Joint Commission, standard nursing care plans and standards of patient teaching, clinical pathways, insurance agency and government payment standards, and utilization review standards. As a result of these standards, hospitals have become centers for managed care and are employing nursing case managers as patient care resource coordinators. All parties involved with health-care delivery, including health-care agencies, health-care providers, insurance companies, and the government, are finding ways to reduce costs while attempting to maintain quality services through managed care.

LEARNING ACTIVITIES

1. Identify the names and locations of books and computer software that contain standardized nursing care plans that you can use as resources for patient care.

2. Locate samples of standards of care at your assigned clinical agency. For discussion, bring to class a standard nursing care plan from a local agency, a clinical pathway, a standardized specific procedure, and patient education materials.

3. Locate the procedure manual from a local health-care agency and compare a procedure you are currently learning from your procedures text to the same procedure in the manual.

4. Identify the person or people at your agency who perform case management, discharge planning, and utilization review. Invite one of them to a clinical post conference to describe their role in decreasing costs while maintaining quality of care in the managed care environment.

REFERENCES

1. U.S. Department of Defense. *Team-STEPPS: Team Strategies and Tools to Enhance Performance and Patient Safety*. Rockville, Md: Agency for Healthcare Research and Quality; 2006. AHRQ publication 06-0020.
2. Institute of Medicine Committee on Quality of Health Care in America. *To Err Is Human: Building a Safer Health System*. Kohn LT, Corrigan JM, Donaldson MS, eds. Washington, DC: National Academy Press; 1999.
3. Schuster PM, Nykolyn L. *Communication for Nurses: How to Prevent Harmful Events and Promote Patient Safety*. Philadelphia, Pa: F.A. Davis; 2010.
4. Schuster PM. Concept maps: Reducing clinical care plan paperwork and increasing learning. *Nurse Educator*. 2000;25(2):76.
5. Novak J, Gowin DB. *Learning How to Learn*. New York, NY: Cambridge University Press; 1984.
6. Ausubel DP, Novak JD, Hanesian H. *Educational Psychology: A Cognitive View*. 2nd ed. New York, NY: Werbel and Peck; 1986.
7. Worrell P. Metacognition: implications for instruction in nursing education. *Journal of Nursing Education*. 1990;29(4):170.
8. All AC, Havens RL. Cognitive/concept map: A teaching strategy for nursing. *Journal of Advanced Nursing*. 1997;25:1210.
9. Baugh NG, Mellott KG: Clinical concept maps as preparation for student nurses' clinical experiences. *Journal of Nursing Education*. 1998;37(6):253.
10. Daley BJ, et al. Concept maps: A strategy to teach and evaluate critical thinking. *Journal of Nursing Education*. 1999;38(1):42.
11. Daley B. Concept maps: linking nursing theory to clinical nursing practice. *Journal of Continuing Education in Nursing*. 1996;27(1):17.
12. Irvine L. Can concept maps be used to promote meaningful learning in nurse education? *Journal of Advanced Nursing*. 1995;21:1175.
13. Kathol DD, et al. Clinical correlation map: a tool for linking theory and practice. *Nurse Educator*. 1998;23(4):31.
14. American Philosophical Association. *Critical Thinking: A Statement of Expert Consensus for Purposes of Educational Assessment and Instruction*. Columbus: Center on Education and Training for Employment, College of Education, The Ohio State University; 1990. ERIC document reproduction no. ED 315-423.
15. McDonald M. Critical thinking. *National League for Nursing Assessment and Evaluation Quarterly*. 2000;1(3).
16. *Nursing: Scope and Standards of Practice*. 2nd ed. Silver Spring, Md: American Nurses Association; 2010. Authored by ANA.
17. Schuster PM. Concept maps in clinical settings: Improved clinical performance and effective patient care. *Dean's Notes*. 2003;25(2).
18. The Joint Commission. Retrieved from http://www.jointcommission.org/cms_renews_joint_commission_hospital_accreditation_deeming_authority/ last accessed September 14, 2014.

2

GATHERING CLINICAL DATA: THE FRAMEWORK FOR CONCEPT CARE MAPPING

OBJECTIVES

1. Identify American Nurses Association (ANA) standards of professional nursing practice and performance for collection of data about the patient's health state and situation.

2. Describe the essential components of a basic patient profile database that are needed to develop a concept care map.

3. Explain the purpose of each component of the basic patient profile database.

4. Identify where to search for clinical data in health-care agencies to develop basic patient profile databases.

5. Identify standardized forms to obtain from the agency that are relevant to a concept care map.

6. Describe how to communicate with staff in the agency when you cannot find clinical data.

Gathering assessment data is the most important thing that student nurses do. This is because each decision regarding patient care is based on clinical data. Sound clinical judgments are based on accurate and complete data collection. The best nurses are excellent at assessment and know why each piece of assessment data is important to the clinical picture.

Many nursing students feel overwhelmed when they arrive at a new clinical unit or agency and try to collect relevant clinical data for their first patient assignments. These same feelings occur each time the student moves to a new agency. As a matter of fact, even experienced nurses feel intimidated by moving from a familiar agency or unit to a new clinical setting, because they fear they may miss important symptoms, which will hinder their ability to make sound clinical judgments.

The purpose of this chapter is to give you guidelines for collecting relevant clinical data based on American Nurses Association (ANA) standards of professional nursing practice and performance. Nursing students are sometimes confused about what is and what is not important clinical data. Therefore, the chapter will describe the reasons why each piece of data is needed, along with where to look for the information that you need to develop a plan of care that is a concept care map. In addition, the chapter outlines the important skill of communicating effectively with staff when you cannot find the information you need to develop a plan of care.

Standards of Professional Performance: Accountability and Responsibility

Nursing students learn early in their nursing programs that they must be accountable and responsible. That is, student nurses are responsible for the nursing care they administer to their assigned patients; they must account for their clinical performance to clinical faculty, who are in turn responsible and accountable for each student. In a clinical agency, the faculty is accountable primarily to the nursing manager when it comes to student activities related to caring for patients. The nurse manager oversees the provision of nursing care.

In addition to being accountable to their faculty, students work directly with and are accountable to agency staff nurses. Agency nurses are responsible for overseeing the care of your patients, and they report directly to the nursing manager. You must know who the staff nurse is for your patient at all times and keep this nurse and your clinical faculty informed of current assessment information. You must tell this nurse what aspects of patient care you will and will not be able to provide to the patient. You must never leave your patients, for a break or any other reason, without giving the staff nurses and your clinical faculty the most recent assessment data for your assigned patients. Communication between you, your faculty, and the staff nurse who is responsible for your assigned patient is critical for safe nursing care of patients.

Student nurses, clinical faculty, and the nursing staff at each agency are legally responsible and accountable. Professional nurses and student nurses may be taken to court and prosecuted for acting in an irresponsible manner. This may sound threatening, but professional nurses and student nurses are responsible and accountable for the care of human beings. Nursing care of patients involves awesome responsibility, with possible legal consequences for negligence when performing outside the standards of professional nursing practice.

Standards of professional nursing practice are inextricably linked to professional accountability and responsibility. You, your faculty, and staff nurses must follow standards of professional practice to act accountably and responsibly. For the purposes of this chapter, we will focus on the first American Nurses Association (ANA) standard of professional nursing practice, which involves the collection of data. Specifically, nurses are responsible for the collection of comprehensive data pertinent to the patient's health and the situation, and that patient data must be documented in a retrievable format.[1]

Data collection occurs *before* development of a plan of care, *before* implementation of nursing care, *during* implementation of nursing care, and *during* evaluation of the patient; therefore, it is continuous. All data must be entered on patient records and be accessible to all health-care providers. The frustrating problem for many students is that they do not know where to look for data in a clinical area. Furthermore, especially early in the nursing education, students typically do not know the most important data to collect. Sometimes students cannot read the writing or understand the abbreviations. Keep in mind that the information exists—you just have to find it. According to ANA standard 1, data must be accessible and recorded. Once you have found the data, of course, you have to know what it means and why it is important.

Finding Important Data

Students are usually given course assessment guidelines to follow when collecting data on patients. A typical example of a patient profile database is found in Figure 2.1. This basic patient profile database has been used to collect data for patients admitted to inpatient or outpatient agencies, such as hospitals or outpatient same-day surgical centers. This assessment tool will serve as the basis of the concept map to be discussed in Chapter 3.

You must know the essential components of a basic patient profile database, the purpose of each component of the profile, and where to search for the information in health-care agencies. This database has physical, psychological, social, and cultural components. Most of the information is collected from patient records, and the remainder may be collected from a brief encounter with your patient and a conversation with the patient's assigned agency nurse. It is best if you can obtain your assignment the evening before clinical, because you have more time to think critically, analyze the data you obtain, and put together a care plan. In outpatient settings, this may not be possible. Students who are unable to obtain an assignment the day before clinical may have to collect data and develop a care plan on the day of care. Each component of the database will be described carefully in the following sections. Refer to Figure 2.1 as you read the remainder of the chapter. Each component of the patient database in Figure 2.1 has been numbered to correspond with the explanations in the following sections.

1) Student Name and Date of Care

Your name and the date of care are needed to help your clinical faculty keep your database separate from those of the other nursing students at your clinical agency.

2) Patient Initials

Never write a patient's full name on anything that will be taken out of the hospital. All information recorded on the patient profile is confidential. Confidentiality involves ethical and legal standards of care. It is your ethical and legal responsibility to reveal confidential information only to health-care professionals directly involved in the patient's care. Be very careful what you do with confidential information: Never leave forms lying

around in patient rooms where the patient, family, or friends may read what you have written, even if you include only initials on the data. Never discuss data with anyone outside the health-care agency.

If a patient's family or friends ask a general question about how the patient is doing, give a general answer, such as "Fine. He's coming along nicely. He ate well and he's up and moving around" or "Not so good today. He's hurting and tired." Do not reveal the specifics of the diagnosis and prognosis. You should tell the inquiring person that the information is confidential, and that specifics should be discussed directly with the patient or with the physician.

3) Age, Growth, and Development

The patient's age can be obtained from the face sheet of the medical record. The face sheet is one of the first few sheets that you will find as you open the medical record; it is the page that is typed by the hospital registration department. On entry to the health-care agency, the first stop the patient makes is the registration desk, where the patient (or a family member) registers for admission.

Age is a very important factor to consider. You must be aware of the human growth and developmental tasks across the life span, and then consider how the current health problem has affected the patient's ability to accomplish the developmental tasks at hand. Erik H. Erikson[2] has a widely known theory of eight stages of human growth and development that you should be familiar with.

Stage 1: *Trust Versus Mistrust*

During the first year of life, infants must learn to trust the people in their environment. When caretakers meet the infants' needs for food, warmth, security, and love, the infants will learn to expect what will happen and to trust those around them to provide for what they need; they feel secure. When infants' needs are not met, the infants become fearful and mistrusting. Some of them fail to thrive. Failure to thrive is a medical condition in which an infant may fail to gain weight or may even lose it. This problem may stem from such environmental causes as physical starvation or emotional deprivation of love and security.

Student Name:

1) Date of Care:	2) Patient Initials:	3) Age: (face sheet)	3) Growth and Development	4) Gender: (face sheet)	5) Admission Date: (face sheet)

6) Reason for hospitalization (face sheet): Describe reason for hospitalization: (expand on back of page) *Medical Dx:* *Pathophysiology:* *All signs and symptoms: Highlight those your patient exhibits*	7) Chronic illnesses (physician's history and physical notes in chart; nursing intake assessment and Kardex)
8) Surgical procedures (consent forms and Kardex): Describe surgical procedure (expand on back of page) Name of surgical procedure: *Describe surgery:*	

9) ADVANCE DIRECTIVES (NURSE'S ADMISSION ASSESSMENTS):

Living will: ☐ Yes ☐ No	Power of attorney: ☐ Yes ☐ No	Do not resuscitate (DNR) order (Kardex): ☐ Yes ☐ No

10) LABORATORY DATA:

Test	Normal Values	Admission	Date/Time	Date/Time	Reason for Abnormal Values
White blood cells (WBCs)					
Red blood cells (RBCs)					
Hemoglobin (Hgb)					
Hematocrit (Hct)					
Platelets					
Prothrombin time (PT)					
International normalized ratio (INR)					
Activated partial thromboplastin time (Aptt)					
Sodium Na					
Potassium K					
Chloride Cl					
Glucose (FBS/BS)					
Hemoglobin A1C					
Cholesterol					
Blood Urea Nitrogen (BUN)					
Creatinine					
Urine analysis (UA)					
Pre-albumin					
Albumin					
Calcium Ca					
Phosphate					
Bilirubin					
Alkaline phosphatase					
SGOT-Serum glutamic-oxyloacetic transaminase					
AST-Serum glutamic pyruvic transaminase					
CK					
CK MB					
Troponin					
B-natriuretic peptide BNP					
pH					
pCO_2					
pO_2					
HCO_3					

11) DIAGNOSTIC TESTS

Chest x-ray:	EKG:	Other abnormal reports:
Sputum or Blood Culture:	Other:	Other:

● Figure 2.1 Patient profile database. Use blue ink for the night before clinical and a different color ink for the day of clinical. Get all of this information the night before clinical, then update it on the day of care.

12) MEDICATIONS

List medications and times of administration (medication administration record and check the drawer in the carts for spelling). Include over-the-counter (OTC) products/herbal medicines.

Times Due				
Brand Name				
Generic Name				
Dose				
Administration Route				
Classification				
Action				
Reason This Patient is Receiving				
Pharmacokinetics	O P D 1/2 M E	O P D 1/2 M E	O P D 1/2 M E	O P D 1/2 M E
Contraindications				
Major Adverse Side Effects				
Nursing Implications				
Pt/Family Teaching				

Developed by P. Testa, YSU

ALLERGIES/PAINS

13) Allergies: Type of Reaction: (medication administration record):	14) When was the last time pain medication given? (medication administration record)
14) Where is the pain? (nurse's notes)	14) How much pain is the patient in on a scale 0-10? (nurse's notes, flow sheet):

TREATMENTS

15) List treatments (Kardex): Rationale for treatments: Dressing changes Ice Foley NG Position changes q2h Ted Hose SCDs IS q1h while awake C&DB q1h while awake etc.
16) Support services (Kardex) What do support services provide for the patient?
17) What does the consultant do for the patient?:

18) DIET/FLUIDS

Type of Diet (Kardex):	Restrictions (Kardex):	Gag reflex intact: ☐Yes ☐No	Appetite: ☐Good ☐Fair ☐Poor	Breakfast ____ %	Lunch ____ %	Dinner ____ %
What type of diet is this?:						
What types of foods are included in this diet and what foods should be avoided?:						

Circle Those Problems That Apply:	
Prior 8 hours Fluid intake: (Oral & IV) Fluid output (flow sheet)	• Problems: swallowing, chewing, dentures (nurse's notes) • Needs assistance with feeding (nurse's notes) • Nausea or vomiting (nurse's notes) • Overhydrated or dehydrated (evaluate total intake and output on flow sheet
Tube feedings: Type and rate (Kardex)	• Belching: • Other:_____

19) INTRAVENOUS FLUIDS (IV therapy record)

Type and Rate:	IV dressing dry, no edema, redness of site: ☐Yes ☐No	Other:

● Figure 2.1 Continued

20) ELIMINATION (flow sheet)

Last bowel movement:	Foley/condom catheter: ☐ Yes ☐ No
Circle Those Problems That Apply:	
• Bowel: constipation, diarrhea, flatus, incontinence, belching • Urinary: hesitancy, frequency, burning, incontinence, odor • Other: _____ • What is causing the problem in elimination? _____	

21) ACTIVITY (Kardex, flow sheet)

Ability to walk (gait):	Type of activity orders:	Use of assistance devices: cane, walker, crutches, prosthesis:	Falls-risk assessment rating:
No. of side rails required (flow sheet)	Restraints (flow sheet): ☐ Yes ☐ No	Weakness ☐ Yes ☐ No	Trouble sleeping (nurse's notes): ☐ Yes ☐ No
What does activity order mean?: _____ Why isn't the patient up ad lib?: _____ Would the problem cause weakness?: _____			

PHYSICAL ASSESSMENT DATA

22) BP (flow sheet):	2) TPR (flow sheet):	23) Height: _____ Weight: _____ (nursing intake assessments)

24) NEUROLOGICAL/MENTAL STATUS:

LOC: alert and oriented to person, place, time (A&O x 3), confused, etc.	Speech: clear, appropriate/inappropriate
Pupils: PERRLA	Sensory deficits for vision/hearing/taste/ smell

25) MUSCULOSKELETAL STATUS:

Bones, joints, muscles (fractures, contractures, arthritis, spinal curvatures, etc):	Extremity (temperature, edema (pitting vs. nonpitting) & sensation)
Motor: ROM x 4 extremities	
Ted hose/plexi pulses/compression devices: type:	Casts, splint, collar, brace:

26) CARDIOVASCULAR SYSTEM:

Pulses (radial, pedal) (to touch or with Doppler):	Capillary refill (< 3s): ☐ Yes ☐ No	
Neck vein (distention):	Sounds: S1, S2, regular, irregular: Apical rate:	Any chest pain:

27) RESPIRATORY SYSTEM:

Depth, rate, rhythm:	Use of accessory muscles:	Cyanosis:	Sputum color, amount:	Cough: productive nonproductive	Breath sounds: clear, rales, wheezes
Use of oxygen: nasal cannula, mask, trach collar:	Flow rate of oxygen:	Oxygen humidification: ☐ Yes ☐ No		Pulse oximeter: _____ % oxygen saturation	Smoking: ☐ Yes ☐ No

28) GASTROINTESTINAL SYSTEM

Abdominal pain, tenderness, guarding; distention, soft, firm:	Bowel sounds x 4 quadrants:	NG tube: describe drainage
Ostomy: describe stoma site and stools:	Other:	

● Figure 2.1 Continued

29) SKIN AND WOUNDS:

Color, turgor: **Pink**	Rash, bruises:	Describe wounds (size, locations):	Edges approximated: ☐ Yes ☐ No	Type of wound drains:
Characteristics of drainage:	Dressings (clean, dry, intact):	Sutures, staples, steri-strips, other:	Risk for pressure ulcer assessment rating:	Other:

30) EYES, EARS, NOSE, THROAT (EENT):

Eyes: redness, drainage, edema, ptosis	Ears: drainage	Nose: redness, drainage, edema	Throat: sore
Psychosocial and Cultural Assessment			
31) Religious preference (face sheet)	32) Marital status (face sheet)	33) Health care benefits and insurance (face sheet):	
34) Occupation (face sheet)	35) Emotional state (nurse's notes)		

● Figure 2.1   Continued

Stage 2: **Autonomy Versus Shame and Doubt**

During the first few years of life, about ages 1 to 3, children explore their surroundings and gain increasing autonomy from their caretakers. Toddlers need much support and encouragement to learn to walk and control bowel and bladder functioning. If parents belittle toddlers, self-doubt and shame occur, and a sense of inferiority may take root.

Stage 3: **Initiative Versus Guilt**

From about ages 3 to 6, children begin to manipulate their environments and become very active. As they take on new challenges successfully with parental support and encouragement, children learn to take the initiative. Lack of parental support and inappropriate scolding for attempts to try new things may lead to feelings of guilt, resentment, and unworthiness.

Stage 4: **Industry Versus Inferiority**

A new stage begins as children enter school and lasts until puberty. Children must learn a new set of social rules as they enter school and develop roles and relationships with teachers and peers outside of their family. Throughout this stage, they must learn to be productive workers at school and at home. Children are expected to develop many self-care skills. They gradually become independent of their families and learn about self-sufficiency. Without parental support, encouragement, and guidance, children may feel inferior and inadequate, and they may lose faith in their own ability to become self-sufficient.

Stage 5: **Ego Identity Versus Role Confusion**

Adolescents are searching for personal identity. Establishing identity involves successful integration of many social roles, such as student, sibling, friend, cheerleader, athlete, band member, or Key Club member. These roles must form coherent patterns that give young people a sense of who they are—their identities. Adolescents need to form close relationships with peers and develop a sexual identity. Their value systems are evolving. They must learn to appreciate their achievements and, toward the end of this stage, select a career. Failure to accomplish this may lead to feelings of hopelessness, despair, and confusion.

Stage 6: **Intimacy Versus Isolation**

The primary task of young adulthood is to love someone else, to form an intimate bond with another person. Failure to accomplish intimacy leads to loneliness. Important tasks include maintaining friendships and establishing new social groups while taking on civic responsibilities in communities. In addition, young adults have the task of growing independent from their parents' home and managing their own households. To do so, they must establish a career. Many choose to marry. Many have their own children and take on parenting roles, which include encouraging and supporting their own children as those children attempt to accomplish the growth and developmental tasks already discussed. In addition, young adults are in the process of formulating a meaningful philosophy of life.

Stage 7: *Generativity Versus Stagnation*

During middle adulthood, the challenge is to remain productive and creative in all aspects of life and to find meaning and joy in careers, family, and community social participation. In contrast to feelings of generativity are feelings of stagnation: Life may become a boring routine, and a person may feel resentful when tasks of this stage are not successfully accomplished. To successfully accomplish this stage of life, individuals may need to review and redirect goals to achieve desired performance in a career. They also may need to develop satisfying hobby and leisure activities.

Middle adults must also accept and adjust to the physical changes of middle age, such as wearing glasses, getting wrinkles, and seeing gray hair. In addition, they need to make adjustments in lifestyles to accommodate aging parents and to maintain relationships with their mates. Those with adolescent children need to assist them in searching for identity and then, as the children leave home, cope with an "empty nest" feeling. As children leave, relationships with spouses are redefined. There may be new roles of in-law and grandparent by the end of this stage.

Stage 8: *Ego Integrity Versus Despair*

During late adulthood, those with a sense of ego integrity have attained an acceptance of their lives and feelings that life has been complete and satisfactory. During this stage, individuals conduct life reviews in which they consider their successes and failures and prepare for the inevitability of death. The task is to make peace with one's self. Although people may not have accomplished everything that they had hoped,

they recognize that it is an imperfect world and that they did the best they could, given the set of circumstances in their lives. They face death without fear, content that they have played a meaningful part in the lives of those around them. In addition, they must continue to affiliate with others the same age while adjusting to the deaths of friends, family members, and spouses.

In contrast to ego integrity is despair. Those in despair believe that too much wrong has occurred and that there is no time to make things better. They may be filled with feelings of resentment, futility, hopelessness, and fear of death.

During this time period, the tasks also include adjusting to changes in physical strength and health, and arranging satisfactory physical living quarters. This includes maintaining a home or apartment, or moving to a retirement center or nursing home. With retirement from the workforce, there is an adjustment to retirement and reduced income. With the loss of work roles, people must find activities that enhance self-worth and usefulness. Some people feel free to pursue whatever activities are important to them. These activities may include a "semiretired" career, a hobby, a sport, or community service activities.

Relevance of Growth and Development to Health State

These eight stages and their associated tasks should be foremost on your mind when you think about your patient's age. A key question is the effect a health problem and its treatment are having and will have on the person's ability to pursue the tasks of a particular age. You can assume that a person's growth and development have been at least temporarily impaired. Depending on the health problem involved, the course of the person's life may be altered permanently. You can also assume that all people entering a health-care setting would rather be doing their life's work and accomplishing the tasks of their age rather than working with you and the other health-care providers to manage health problems. The challenge to nurses is to get patients back on track and to promote optimal levels of growth and development or a peaceful death.

4) Gender

Look at the face sheet to find the patient's gender. It is important that you be aware of gender differences in communication and that you communicate clearly with both sexes. Specifically, women tend to be focused on affiliation through communication, wanting to establish intimacy and form communal connections. In contrast, men tend to be focused on attaining independence and status through communication and are concerned with hierarchy in human relationships. These differing gender goals influence the nature of human relationships, including the relationships between health-care providers and patients. For example, to some men, illness may be viewed as taking away independence and status, resulting in feelings of powerlessness. But women who are functioning with affiliation goals in mind may willingly accept the support of health-care providers. As you perform assessments, be aware of gender differences in communication so that you can clearly decipher messages from patients of both sexes.[3,4]

5) Admission Date

Look on the face sheet for the patient's admission date. It is important to know how long the person has been in the health-care system. With managed care, there is usually a specific amount of time allotted to each type of problem; for example, a patient having knee replacement is in the hospital for 3 to 4 days. You can begin to determine if your patient is on or off the expected course of treatment just by knowing the date of admission and the expected length of stay for the type of problem the patient was admitted for.

6) Reason for Hospitalization

The reason for hospitalization is typed clearly on the face sheet, without abbreviations. Many students struggle with abbreviations and poor handwriting, which can be avoided by obtaining the reason for hospitalization from the face sheet. This is generally a medical diagnosis and, if applicable, includes the surgical procedure. Although many things may have happened to a patient during hospitalization, it is important to know what the initial problem was that brought the person into the hospital.

7) Chronic Illnesses

The face sheet contains information on past and present chronic illnesses in addition to the reason for hospitalization. It is important to note chronic illnesses that are listed as medical diagnoses in the physician's history and progress notes. This information on chronic illness is also found on the nurse's initial intake history and physical assessment forms. These are located in the patient's medical record. Many facilities—but not all—summarize pertinent information on a Kardex. The Kardex is a quick reference for nurses that contains critical information for the most current care of the patient. Facilities that use a Kardex may have slight variations in format; however, the information contained on it is almost universal.

You must look up each chronic illness and current medical diagnosis in your pathophysiology book, which will have the most complete definitions of the diseases, with pathological effects and etiologies. Highlight all the signs and symptoms your patient exhibits at the present time. It is not at all uncommon for the same patient to have a number of chronic conditions that are different from the reason for admission. For example, a patient may have chronic diabetes and hypertension but be currently admitted for a small bowel obstruction. All medical problems must be identified and defined, because in order to develop the nursing care plan you must have a clear picture of the clinical problems that may occur.

8) Surgical Procedures

The best place to find out what types of surgical procedures the patient has undergone (or is about to undergo) is the surgical consent forms in the patient's medical record. This is because legal standards demand that the exact procedure be specified and that no abbreviations be used. The surgical procedure is also listed on the Kardex, but it may be abbreviated there and therefore more difficult to interpret.

When trying to understand the nature of the surgical procedures, you can start with a medical dictionary for a basic definition. However, the best reference is a nursing medical-surgical text with more detailed descriptions of surgical procedures. Sometimes you can find typed surgical operative notes, dictated by the surgeon and transcribed by people in the medical records department, but this is not usually available in the medical record until a few days after surgery.

9) Advance Directives

This information is found on the admission nurse's assessment form; it should also appear on the Kardex. Health-care facilities are required by law to ask patients if they have advance directives, which are legal documents such as a living will or a health-care power of attorney. A living will outlines the patient's wishes about life-sustaining treatments; typically, it tells health-care providers to withhold life-sustaining treatments if the patient has a terminal condition and cannot make his own decisions. A health-care power of attorney appoints a person to make health-care decisions on the patient's behalf if the patient is unable to do so.

DNR is a crucial abbreviation to remember. It stands for *do not resuscitate*. If the patient has a DNR order, it will be listed on the Kardex, sometimes with a red label on the outside of the chart. It means that the person does not want cardiopulmonary resuscitation (CPR) or other extreme measures performed if he/she goes into cardiac or respiratory arrest. The person may be given drugs and kept comfortable and the goal is a peaceful death with dignity.

10) Laboratory Data

A specific section of the medical record is set aside for the patient's laboratory values.[5] Results of the blood and urine tests described in the following sections are important to know for any patient, whether the values are normal or abnormal. Many additional tests may be ordered based on the pathophysiology of the patient's disease. Of course, all currently abnormal results are very important, because they reveal the extent of disease.

Make sure you know which tests are ordered for your clinical day of care, because intravenous (IV) fluids and medication administration are directly linked to what is happening in the patient's blood and urine. You must check the new daily laboratory values before giving IV fluids and medications; for example, if you are giving insulin at 8 a.m., make sure you know the blood glucose value from the 6 a.m. draw. If the blood glucose value is too low, the insulin may be held (see Table 2.1). Likewise, if you are giving enoxaparin sodium (Lovenox) at 8 a.m., make sure you know results of the patient's platelet test before you give the medication. The dose of enoxaparin (Lovenox) will be held if platelets drop too low.

You should know the values of your patient's blood for the following commonly ordered blood and urine tests. These tests are universally ordered on almost all patients and serve as a baseline assessment for planning nursing care.

Inflammation and Infection: White Blood Cells

The abbreviation for white blood cells is WBCs. As a rule of thumb, the white blood cell count should be less than $10,000/mm^3$. An elevated white blood cell count indicates inflammation and infection. The white blood cells may be broken down into a differential count of each cell type. An increase in the number of neutrophils (band and stab cells) indicates an acute infection, also known as a *"shift to the left."* Other types of white blood cells (basophils and eosinophils) are elevated in allergic reactions. Still others are lymphocytes, involved in developing immunity, and phagocytic monocytes that engulf bacteria. A low white blood cell count (below $5000/mm^3$) indicates problems in producing cells from the bone marrow, which may happen during chemotherapy.

Anemia and Bleeding: Red Blood Cells, Hemoglobin, and Hematocrit

For detecting disorders such as anemia, red blood cells (RBCs) are normally at around 5.4 million/mcL for men and 4.8 million/mcL for women. Hemoglobin (Hgb) and Hematocrit (Hct) are commonly abbreviated as H&H. Hemoglobin is a reflection of the concentration of red blood cells in the blood, usually 14 to 18 g/dL in male patients and 12 to 16 g/dL in female patients. The main reason that the hemoglobin level drops is bleeding. When the hemoglobin level drops below 9 g/dL, blood transfusions may be required.

Hematocrit is the percentage of red blood cells in the total blood volume. The total blood volume consists of red blood cells and serum. In male patients, a normal hematocrit level is 42% to 52%. In female patients, a normal hematocrit level is 37% to 47%. The hematocrit level should be about three times the hemoglobin concentration. When the patient is bleeding, the hematocrit will drop along with the hemoglobin level. Hematocrit also reflects the patient's state of hydration; when the patient is dehydrated, the hemoglobin level will be normal or slightly high and the hematocrit will be low.

Blood Coagulation Studies

Blood coagulation studies include platelet counts, international normalized ratio (INR), prothrombin time (PT), partial thromboplastin time (PTT), and activated partial thromboplastin time (APTT).

Platelets

Platelets are thrombocytes, which are cells essential to blood clotting. The normal platelet count is between 150,000 and 400,000/mm³. The platelet count typically decreases because of bleeding; and certain drugs can also hinder the bone marrow in its production of these cells. For example, enoxaparin (Lovenox), which is used to prevent formation of blood clots in the legs in immobilized patients, has a side effect of decreasing platelets. For that reason, platelet counts are monitored during enoxaparin (Lovenox) administration. The drug is usually discontinued when platelets drop below 130,000/mm³.

INR, PT, PTT, and APTT

Values for international normalized ratio (INR), prothrombin time (PT) (sometimes called *pro time*), partial thromboplastin time (PTT), and activated partial thromboplastin time (APTT) reflect different ways to express the time it takes for blood to coagulate and clot. The therapeutic international normalized ratio (INR) for treatment has a range of 2.0 to 3.0, prothrombin time (PT) is normally 11 to 12.5 seconds, partial thromboplastin time (PTT) is normally 60 to 70 seconds, and activated partial thromboplastin time (APTT) is normally 30 to 40 seconds. Although these values all reflect blood clotting

ability, they differ somewhat: partial thromboplastin time (PTT) and activated partial thromboplastin time (APTT) are used to assess the intrinsic system of clotting, while prothrombin time (PT) and international normalized ratio (INR) are used to assess the extrinsic system of clotting. These values are very important because many patients take anticoagulants to increase the time it takes for a clot to form. For example, immobilized patients are routinely placed on anticoagulation therapy to prevent formation of blood clots. Partial thromboplastin time (PTT) or activated partial thromboplastin time (APTT) is used to assess the effects of the anticoagulant heparin, which is given subcutaneously or intravenously. The prothrombin time or international normalized ratio (INR) is used to assess the effect of the anticoagulant warfarin (Coumadin), which is given orally. Heparin affects the intrinsic system of clotting, and warfarin (Coumadin) affects the extrinsic system of clotting.

In either case, patients receiving anticoagulant therapy will have purposely prolonged clotting times that are 1.5 to 2.5 times the control value. Heparin and warfarin (Coumadin) dosages are regulated up or down to maintain the anticoagulation at 1.5 to 2.5 times the control value. Therefore, you must know the patient's latest international normalized ratio (INR) or prothrombin time (PT) before giving warfarin (Coumadin), the latest activated partial thromboplastin time (APTT) or partial thromboplastin time (PTT) before giving heparin, and the latest platelet count before giving enoxaparin (Lovenox).

Electrolytes and Cellular Functioning

Probably the most important electrolyte to be aware of is potassium. The normal potassium level is about 3.5 to 5.5 mEq/L. Too much or too little of this electrolyte will have profound effects on all muscles, but of particular concern is the heart muscle. The ability of the heart to contract and the rate at which it contracts depend on normal potassium levels. Potassium levels typically decline with vomiting and diarrhea. Potassium-depleting diuretics are another common cause of decreased potassium levels.

Potassium is commonly added to intravenous (IV) fluids and given in oral preparations. Make sure you know the patient's latest potassium levels before giving potassium supplements, either intravenously or orally. In addition, patients taking digitalis (Lanoxin) may develop toxic levels of the drug in their bloodstream when potassium levels are too low, inducing serious cardiac arrhythmias.

There are a few other important electrolytes to monitor. For example, serum sodium (135 to 145 mEq/L) and chloride (97 to 107 mEq/L) are important in the regulation of water balance and pH. Calcium (8.2 to 10.2 mg/dL) and phosphorus (2.5 to 4.5mg/dL) are important for bone strength and muscle functioning (including the heart muscle).

All electrolytes must be balanced carefully through appropriate oral nutrition and oral vitamin and mineral supplementation. If the patient is not able to ingest or digest the appropriate foods, then intravenous (IV) therapy will be instituted to maintain fluid and electrolyte balance.

Nutrition: Blood Glucose, Glycosylated Hemoglobin, and Cholesterol

Tests of blood glucose, glycosylated hemoglobin, and cholesterol are used to assess a patient's current glucose level and long-term glucose control.

Blood Glucose
The level of glucose in a patient's blood after fasting (also known as the *fasting blood sugar*) is normally 70 to 110 mg/dL. Persistently elevated blood glucose levels may indicate diabetes mellitus. Because diabetes is so common, this is a common test.

Typically, when the blood glucose level is too low, the cause is unintentional insulin overdose. Consider this example: A patient's 6 a.m. glucose level is within normal limits, so the nurse gives the patient's 7 a.m. insulin, thinking that the patient will be eating breakfast. But the patient begins feeling nauseated and does not eat. In this case, expect an insulin reaction, because the blood glucose is guaranteed to drop.

Patients who are "brittle," which means that their blood glucose is not under control and can fluctuate widely, should be checked in the morning, usually around 6 a.m. The result of this test is the fasting blood glucose. Nonfasting blood glucose levels are commonly checked before lunch,

before supper, and at bedtime. In brittle diabetics, insulin is given on a sliding scale based on the blood glucose readings (see Table 2.1).

Glycosylated Hemoglobin
Glycosylated hemoglobin (also called *glycohemoglobin*) is another common test of blood glucose. It is used to measure long-term blood glucose control over a period of up to 120 days. Glucose binds to hemoglobin in a chemical reaction. When the patient is diabetic and blood glucose levels are elevated, the percentage of glycosylated hemoglobin is higher. This reaction is not reversible; once the glycogen attaches, it remains with the red blood cell for its life cycle, about 120 days. Therefore, you can tell if the patient's blood glucose has been under control over time. Normal, healthy people have 5.5% to 8.8% of total hemoglobin bound to glucose. Diabetics under control range from 7.5% to 11.4% total hemoglobin bound to glucose, whereas those who need either more diet instruction or more insulin (or both) will be higher. There are actually three types of hemoglobin that become glycosylated: A1a, A1b, and A1c. Many laboratories report only the A1c level, which is normally 3.56% bound to glucose.[5]

Cholesterol
The cholesterol level indicates the amount of lipids or fats in the blood. Lipids are carried in the blood in combination with proteins, and are thus called lipoproteins. High levels of cholesterol are a risk factor for cardiovascular disease, which is the primary health problem in the United States. Numerous people have cholesterol levels above 200 mg/dL. Cholesterol is composed of high-density lipoproteins (HDLs), low-density lipoproteins (LDLs), and triglycerides.

Table 2.1	Sliding Scale Insulin Dosages*	
Blood Glucose Level	Insulin Dosage
151–200 mg/dL	6 units
201–250 mg/dL	8 units
251–300 mg/dL	10 units
301–400 mg/dL	12 units

*Sample guidelines for regular sliding scale insulin. The higher the blood glucose, the more insulin needed to regulate blood glucose levels.

Of primary interest in relation to cardiac disease are the low density lipoproteins (LDLs), which should be below 130 mg/dL. Low density lipoproteins have been called "bad" cholesterol because they produce atherosclerosis. Many people take lipid lowering drugs such as atorvastatin calcium (Lipitor) to reduce their levels of low density lipoproteins. They also are prescribed a low cholesterol diet and an exercise program.

Kidney Functioning

Blood urea nitrogen and creatinine levels are commonly used to determine the functioning of the kidneys. Normal creatinine values are below 1.5 mg/dL, while blood urea nitrogen ranges between 8 and 23 mg/dL.

Urinalysis is done mainly to check for infection and to check kidney function. Bladder infections are extremely common, especially in women, because they have a shorter urethra than men. Typically, a clean catch urine specimen is obtained. The patient wipes the urethra with special antiseptic solution, voids a little in the toilet, and then inserts a sterile cup under the urine stream until the cup contains about 30 mL. This specimen should contain fewer than 10,000 bacteria/mL, provided the patient has wiped the urethra properly to decrease the number of normal flora around the meatus. A specimen obtained from a sterile catheterization, where a sterile tube is inserted into the sterile bladder, should contain no bacteria. In addition, the urine should contain no protein, blood, ketones, or glucose. Any of these substances in urine usually indicates diabetes or kidney disease.

Liver Functioning

Bilirubin is the product of the breakdown of RBCs by the liver. Normal values are 0.3 to 1.1 mg/dL. With liver failure, bilirubin levels rise and the patient becomes jaundiced as a result. There are three important liver enzymes: alkaline phosphatase (ALP), normally 35 to142 U/L in males and 25 to125 U/L in females; aspartate aminotransferase (AST), normally 19 to 48 U/L in males and 9 to 36 U/L in females; and alanine aminotransferase (ALT), normally 10 to 40 U/L in males and 7 to 35 U/L in females. These values will all be elevated with liver disease, such as hepatitis, cirrhosis, or liver failure. A functioning liver is crucial to the metabolism of drugs, and many drugs can be damaging to the liver, so monitoring liver function is very important.

Heart Functioning

There are blood studies to analyze the functioning of the heart; for example, tests to diagnose myocardial infarction include blood levels of creatine kinase (CK), normally 38 to174 U/L in males and 26 to140 U/L in females. CK-MB, specific to myocardial cells, is normally less than 4% to 6% of the total creatine kinase (CK) value. Elevated creatine kinase (CK) indicates damage to myocardial cells during acute myocardial infarction. Creatine kinase (CK) is an enzyme that is released into the serum from damaged myocardial cells within the first 48 hours, and CK-MB's appear in the first 6 to 24 hours. With heart muscle damage, troponin I (normally below 0.35 ng/ml) and troponin T (normally below 0.20 ug/L) will be elevated between 2 and 6 hours after myocardial infarction. In addition, B-type natriuretic peptide (BNP) serum values (normally below 100 pg/mL) increase proportional to the degree of congestive heart failure. B-type natriuretic peptide (BNP) is produced in the left ventricle with increased ventricular pressure and volume of blood in the ventricle, which are the result of heart failure.

Respiratory Functioning and Acid Base Balance

Blood gases are analyzed whenever respiratory functioning is of concern and the patient may not be getting enough oxygen. An arterial blood sample is obtained to determine the amount of oxygen in the blood (PO_2); it is normally 80 to 95 mm Hg and will be decreased without adequate respirations. In addition, carbon dioxide levels (PCO_2), normally 35 to 45 mm Hg, will rise without adequate respirations. As the patient lacks oxygen and becomes hypoxic, he becomes acidic, and the blood pH (normally 7.35 to 7.45) will decrease. In addition, bicarbonate (HCO_3), normally 18 to 23 mEq/L is also measured. In response to respiratory acidosis (which is due to respiratory failure), the kidneys will retain the base bicarbonate to compensate for the acidosis, so bicarbonate levels will rise.

Always record any recent abnormal laboratory values (within 1 day of your clinical assignment), and the laboratory values on admission. Laboratory reports are very important in determining the extent of the patient's chronic and acute diseases and the outcomes of surgery, such as the amount of blood lost during surgery, or the patient's bleeding after surgery. Medication administration and medical treatments are based on the results of analysis of blood. The goal will be to develop a care map that reflects the coordination of pathology and assessment data with laboratory data, medications, and treatments used to control chronic and acute responses to health problems.

11) Diagnostic Tests

Your patient may undergo a wide range of diagnostic tests. Perhaps the two most common tests are a chest x-ray and an electrocardiogram (EKG).

Chest X-ray

You can find chest x-ray reports in the patient's medical record with the laboratory and diagnostic procedures. The chest x-ray is a basic diagnostic test used to examine the structure of the heart and lungs. Enlargement of the heart and areas of lung consolidation, which could result from pneumonia or tumors, can be detected on chest x-rays.

Electrocardiogram

The electrocardiogram (EKG) indicates patterns of electrical activity and contraction of the heart muscle. This test is routinely performed on patients over age 35 as part of a general physical examination. The report is also found with the laboratory and diagnostic procedures in the patient's medical record. Although student nurses are not expected to interpret electrocardiogram tracings, the interpretation is printed on the report along with the rhythm strips indicating the rate and rhythm of the heart.

Sputum and Blood Cultures

Sputum specimens coughed up from the lungs are used to determine the type of microorganism that is causing an infection of the lungs. Blood cultures are obtained when the patient is believed to be septic because an infecting organism has spread systemically throughout the body. Sputum or blood specimens are smeared on a culture plate and incubated to grow the bacteria. Then bacteria are examined under a microscope, and the types of drugs that may be used to kill the organism are determined.

12) Medications

One of the most important, and dangerous, tasks nurses are responsible for is medication administration. This includes all drugs the patient is taking, prescriptions as well as over-the-counter (OTC) and herbal medications. From virtually the first day of classes, nurses learn the six "rights" of drug administration:

- Right drug
- Right patient
- Right dose
- Right route
- Right time
- Right to refuse a medication

This sounds simple enough, but despite the best intentions of nurses and other health-care professionals, medication errors occur. They can harm or kill patients. Consequently, you must be exceedingly careful whenever you work with medications.

To find information about your patient's medications, look on the medication sheet, also known as the *medication record,* which usually is kept in the same place as the Kardex. List each drug and the times it should be administered on your patient profile database. Sometimes drugs are misspelled on these sheets; therefore, you should go directly to the patients' medication drawer or wherever drugs are kept and copy the name and dosage of the drug from the paper wrapper on the drug. That way, you can be sure you have spelled the drug name correctly.

When you get home, you will need to look up and study each drug. You may want to consider purchasing a drug book or set of drug cards so you can highlight important actions and side effects.

Computer programs are also available, and they save time in finding drug information. Also consider looking on the Internet for drug information. Keep in mind that not every drug is available in a given drug reference. Be very careful that you have a valid and reliable source of information when obtaining information from the Internet.

If you are unable to find a drug in your reference book or computer program, call the pharmacy at the health-care institution or the pharmacist at the local drug store. Tell the pharmacist that you are a nursing student and would like information on a drug. For example, suppose you cannot find Alu-Tab tablets in your drug cards. Ask the pharmacist to give you information about that drug over the phone.

As you research your drugs, always write down the times the drug is to be administered and the brand or trade name and generic name of the drug. Many times the brand or trade name is listed on a medication record but a generic drug is substituted by the pharmacy. Sometimes, two generic drugs will be substituted for a single combination trade name drug. This may seem very confusing at first. For example, the trade name drug Diovan HCT contains both valsartan and hydrochlorothiazide in one tablet. The pharmacy may substitute two generic tablets, one tablet of valsartan and one tablet of hydrochlorothiazide. Substitutions are made by pharmacies to decrease the cost associated with brand name drugs. You must know the composition of each tablet to be administered, and you must be especially careful when combination drugs have been ordered.

You must know the dose to be administered and whether the dose is within the range recommended by the drug's manufacturer. Also identify how the drug is to be administered, also known as the *route of administration*. Be sure that the dose of the drug is compatible with the route of administration.

It is most important to recognize the general classification to which any particular drug belongs. This will help you in identifying where the drug belongs on the care map. For example:

▶ Antibiotics are grouped with the nursing diagnosis related to an infection or potential for infection, such as ***Impaired Urinary Elimination*** if the patient has a urinary tract infection.

▶ Antidysrhythmics and antihypertensives are grouped with ***Decreased Cardiac Output.***

▶ Anticoagulants and diuretics are grouped with ***Deficient Fluid Volume.***

▶ Corticosteroids are grouped with ***Ineffective Protection.***

▶ Anticonvulsants are grouped with ***Risk for Ineffective Cerebral Tissue Perfusion.***

▶ Insulins are grouped with ***Imbalanced Nutrition: Less Than Body Requirements.***

▶ Drugs used for pain are grouped with ***Acute Pain*** or ***Chronic Pain.***

You must determine the actions of each drug. Many times there is more than one action of a drug; in that case, identify the specific reason your patient is receiving the drug. For example, determine whether your patient is taking aspirin to relieve pain, to bring down a temperature, or as an anticoagulant.

You must be aware of the pharmacokinetics of medications, including the onset (O), peak (P), duration (D), and half-life (1/2) of each drug. In addition, find out how the drug is metabolized (M) and excreted (E) by the body. Many drugs are metabolized in the liver and excreted by the kidneys. Therefore, you must know the status of liver and renal functioning through analysis of laboratory data as described previously.

Contraindications for drugs are also important. Under what conditions should the patient not be taking the drug? What are the major adverse effects or side effects of each drug? Every drug has side effects that must be carefully monitored in patients. For example, the side effects of many antibiotics include nausea and diarrhea.

Nursing implications include what the nurse should assess while the patient is taking the drug. If a patient is on a blood pressure medication, the nurse should know what the patient's blood pressure is before administering the drug. If the nurse is administering potassium, the nurse should know the potassium level. In addition, there is patient and family teaching to be done with each drug. The patient must be taught everything he needs to know to take care of himself at home if he is to be discharged with the drug, and at least the purpose of the drug to be administered while he/she is hospitalized.

13) Allergies

Allergies to drugs may appear in many places in patient records. Allergies are critical to note, because an allergic reaction may lead to anaphylactic shock and death. In many institutions, the front of the chart itself will have a red label on it noting drug allergies. The medication record will have a space for drug allergies, and the Kardex will also list drug allergies.

14) Pain Medications and Pain Ratings

Pain control is always a priority in the patient plan of care. Find out when the patient last received a pain medication, what type of medication it was, and the dosage administered. You can find this information on the medication administration record. Look at the pattern of pain medication administration. This will give you an indication of the amount of pain the patient has been experiencing. Keep in mind, though, that not all patients will ask for pain medication, even when they are uncomfortable.

Pain Ratings

A patient's perception of pain is documented on flow sheets and on the nurses' notes. (Flow sheets are a special form of nurses' notes used to record routine observations.) Patients are usually asked to rate the amount of pain they feel on a scale from 0 to 10, with 0 as no pain and 10 as the worst pain ever experienced. You need to locate the most recent pain rating on the nurses' notes. Subjective pain ratings can be used in addition to the data collected about the patient's use of pain medications. In addition, the location of the patient's pain is also recorded.

15) Treatments and Their Relation to Medical and Nursing Diagnoses

Examples of patient treatments include oxygen administration, incentive spirometry, catheterization, nasogastric intubation, and dressing changes. These are all the things being done to the patient. You will eventually be responsible for ensuring that all treatments are done. The treatments are listed on the Kardex. It is important to note what these treatments are, even if you have not yet learned how to do them all. Your agency nurse may actually perform a treatment that you have not yet learned how to do.

You must know the rationale for each of the treatments. Look up and define each treatment, and know why the patient is receiving the treatment as it relates to the medical and nursing diagnoses. For example, the patient may be instructed to do incentive spirometry breathing exercises every hour while awake, to promote deep breathing and oxygenation in the lungs and to prevent pneumonia. Treatments are written on the map under the appropriate nursing diagnoses; for example, the incentive spirometry may be listed under the nursing diagnosis of **Impaired Gas Exchange**.

16) Support Services

Support services are all the disciplines involved in the patient's care. Professionals in these disciplines include dietitians, physical and occupational therapists, speech and respiratory therapists, and social workers. It is important to identify the role of each discipline in the patient's care. The nurse's role is to assess the patient's health state and to recognize whether the patient will be able to tolerate the services that are scheduled. The nurse then communicates as appropriate with the support services and the attending physician, and gives recommendations for therapy.

For example, a patient is supposed to be ambulated in the hall post-operatively after a total hip replacement. You know that the patient's morning hemoglobin was 8 g/dL, the patient is scheduled for a transfusion, her blood pressure was lower than it was yesterday, her face is pale, and her nail beds are white. You are responsible for discussing patient data with the physical therapist and recommending that the patient be exercised in bed and ambulated to a chair, and that the physical therapist should wait until after the transfusion to get the patient up and walking in the hall.

In another example, the patient has asthma and receives inhalation treatments every 4 hours. You note that the patient's breathing is worsening even though the 4 hours have not elapsed. You should intervene and call the respiratory therapist to report the problem and ask if the therapist could arrive right on time or even a few minutes early for the next treatment.

17) Consultations

Consultants are physicians who are specialists, such as cardiologists, pulmonologists, and gastroenterologists. They are also listed on the Kardex and in the patient's medical record. The primary doctor who admitted the patient to the hospital will call in a specialist when the doctor suspects that the patient's medical problem resides in a specific organ system. In essence, the primary doctor is asking the opinion and treatment advice of the specialist. If you know the specialty of the consultants, you know which physiological components of the body to assess most carefully, because the primary physician would not need the services of the consultant unless something was likely to be wrong with that

system of the body. Consultants typically focus on one body system.

18) Type of Diet

The type of diet the patient is following and any dietary restrictions are always listed on the Kardex. The nursing diagnosis ***Imbalanced Nutrition: Less Than Body Requirements*** is very common, and patients often have knowledge deficits and problems in managing and adhering to prescribed diets. A regular or general diet is based on the MyPlate guidelines issued by the U.S. government and shown in Figure 2.2. The most common types of special and restricted diets are described next.

NPO—Nothing by Mouth

Many patients are NPO (*nulla/nil/non per os*) for surgery or for diagnostic testing, to prevent aspiration during procedures.

● Figure 2.2 MyPlate nutrition guidelines.

Liquid Diet

After surgery or tests for which the patient has been NPO, she may receive clear liquids because they are easy to digest. Also, surgical patients who may be nauseated by anesthesia and pain medications tolerate clear liquids best. The clear liquid diet is missing many nutrients, but it does provide fluids.

Clear liquids are anything that you can see through, such as tea, 7-Up, apple juice, Sprite, ginger ale, Popsicles, Jell-O, sherbet, and broth. Orange juice and coffee, two of the most common drinks, should be avoided by nauseated patients because they are acidic and likely to induce vomiting. As nausea improves, the patient can be advanced to full liquids, which includes milk, ice cream, fruit juices, and cooked cereals.

Soft Diet

A soft diet is commonly prescribed for stroke patients, patients without teeth, and patients who have had throat surgery—in short, for anyone who has trouble chewing or swallowing. Stroke patients have trouble chewing and swallowing because of paralysis. After throat surgery, patients may have problems swallowing because of pain. To make a soft diet, regular foods from the myplate guidelines can be put into a food processor and pureed. Patients at home may opt to buy strained baby food from the grocery store.

Low-Fat Diet

A low-fat diet may be recommended for patients with cardiovascular disease, hypertension, or gallbladder disease. In cardiovascular disease, low-fat diets are recommended to decrease high cholesterol levels. Low-fat diets are also used to control gallbladder spasm in gallbladder disease, since fat in the intestines prompts the gallbladder to release bile to digest the fat. If the gallbladder ducts are obstructed by stones or other pathology, gallbladder spasms can be very painful and cause what is commonly called a *gallbladder attack*.

Low-Sodium Diet

Patients with cardiovascular disease are commonly put on low-sodium diets to reduce fluid retention, because anywhere sodium goes, water always follows. Cardiac patients commonly retain fluids, so limited amounts of sodium are allowed in the diet to promote excretion of extra fluids. Sometimes cardiac patients are also placed on fluid restrictions.

Low-Protein Diet

Low-protein diets are common among patients with liver and kidney failure. The liver normally metabolizes protein breakdown products, such as nitrogenous ammonia. Without conversion of ammonia to urea for excretion by the kidneys, ammonia levels build in the blood. Ammonia crosses the blood brain barrier and results in encephalopathy (malfunction of the brain), in which the patient will have symptoms such as disorientation, decreased levels of consciousness, and sensory deficits.

Low-protein diets are also common in renal failure, because the kidneys are unable to excrete urea. Although the liver is functioning and produces urea, the kidneys can no longer excrete it. Thus, levels of blood urea nitrogen (BUN) increase, urea crosses the blood brain barrier, and encephalopathy results.

Low-Sugar Diet

Diabetic patients are unable to break down sugar (glucose) for use by any cells of the body. That means diabetics can eat very little candy, cake, pie, or other foods that contain high concentrations of sugar. Diabetes is treated by controlling the total amount of calories along with the portions of protein, fat, and carbohydrates in all food taken into the body.

Food intake must be regulated in conjunction with the quantity of insulin given, as well as the amount of daily exercise activities. Diabetics must learn to eat balanced meals and snacks that contain healthy foods low in sugar and cholesterol. Food exchange lists are based on the myplate guidelines as shown in Figure 2.2. These lists show what counts as a serving of meat, fruit, milk, vegetables, or fat. For a sample daily menu, the patient may be told to eat:

- 1 fruit, 2 breads, 1 milk, and 1 teaspoon of fat for breakfast

- ▶ 2 ounces of meat, 3 breads, 1 teaspoon of fat, 1 vegetable, and 1 fruit for lunch
- ▶ 3 ounces of meat, 2 breads, 2 teaspoons of fat, and 2 vegetables for supper
- ▶ A snack of 1 milk, 1 bread, and 1 teaspoon of fat

Weight Reduction Diet

Weight reduction diets control calories while still providing all the nutrients essential for health. Healthy weight reduction diets use food exchange lists in a manner very similar to diabetic diets, balancing fruits, breads, vegetables, meats, and fats consumed during each meal. Weight reduction diets should not go below 1200 calories a day, because it is nearly impossible to obtain the essential nutrients needed each day in less than 1200 calories.

Food is fuel for the body. Every activity requires fuel to produce energy. To lose weight, patients must burn more calories than they consume. The loss of 1 pound requires burning 3500 calories more than are consumed. Exercise is an important component of any weight reduction plan. The patient will increase the amount of energy used by burning more calories through exercise, thus improving weight loss. Added benefits from exercise include improved muscle tone and overall stamina. A health goal is to gradually build up to walking a minimum of 30 minutes a day, at least 4 days a week.

High-Fiber Diet

High-fiber diets are typically recommended to promote healthy bowel functioning and normal bowel movements. High-fiber foods include whole grain or bran breads and cereals, and foods with skins or seeds.

Low-Residue Diet

Patients with inflammatory bowel disease such as colitis, enteritis, or Crohn's disease commonly cannot tolerate foods high in fiber. These patients are placed on low-residue diets. *Residue* refers to the indigestible substances left in the gastrointestinal tract after digestion and absorption have occurred. With inflammation of the bowel, fibrous foods can be irritating and cause pain. Low residue foods are mild in flavor, well cooked, and tender. Tender cuts of meat, canned fruits, cottage cheese, and white low-fiber breads are examples of foods in this diet.

Bland Diet

Sometimes patients with gastrointestinal or bowel problems may be placed on bland diets, which are chemically and mechanically nonstimulating. Thus, these diets include bland and soft foods.

Tube Feeding

A patient who can digest food but cannot chew or swallow may receive food through a tube threaded into the stomach. This is called tube feeding. The tube may be passed from the nose to the stomach (nasogastric or NG tube), or it may be surgically inserted through the abdominal wall and into the stomach (gastric or G-tube).

A liquid food formula that contains all nutrients needed to maintain health is infused down the tube directly to the patient's stomach, bypassing the throat to avoid aspiration. The patient may have a continuous feeding, with a machine continually pumping formula at a specific hourly rate, or the patient may receive bolus feedings, in which a specific amount of formula is given all at one time. The patient typically receives a bolus at breakfast, lunch, dinner, and bedtime.

The type or brand of tube feeding, and the amount to be infused in milliliters per hour or the amount to be given in a bolus will appear in the Kardex, under diet. Also, go to the patient's room or the kitchen and look at the cans of formula; record the amount of protein, fat, and carbohydrate in each can. There are many types of food formulas designed to meet patients' special dietary needs. For example, special tube feeding formulas have been manufactured to contain reduced protein or partially digested protein for patients who have renal failure or liver failure.

Priority Nutrition Assessments

Nutritional assessments are especially important for patients who are confused or paralyzed or have decreased levels of consciousness. They will need assistance with eating, and calorie counts may be required to track daily intake of food and fluids to ensure adequate nutritional intake. These patients have trouble putting food to their mouths, chewing it, or swallowing it. If a patient cannot chew or swallow, she may choke and aspirate food into the lungs. For example, a patient who has had a stroke may be paralyzed on one side of her mouth and throat and may have decreased levels of consciousness.

Perform a careful assessment for a patient who has had his throat numbed, because he will be temporarily unable to swallow. For example, following a bronchoscopy or endoscopy procedure, the gag reflex is temporarily paralyzed to facilitate passage of the tube into the lungs, stomach, or small intestine. Never feed someone after such a procedure until you check to make sure the gag reflex has returned. As you consider the patient's diagnosis and procedures, always consider the effect on the patient's ability to move his arms and place food into his own mouth, as well as his ability to swallow and chew.

The patient's appetite and amount of food consumed are usually listed as a specific percentage of food eaten off a tray, such as *50% of breakfast, 25% of lunch,* and *100% of supper.* The amount of food consumed is generally found on the nursing flow sheets. Flow sheets are used to record routine observations such as diet. In addition, any record of problems with nausea, vomiting, or diarrhea will be found in the nurses' notes.

Many patients have problems with fluid balance and need to have their fluid intake and urinary output monitored to track the milliliters of fluid taken in and the amount of urine output and other drainages during each shift. Fluid intake and output for each shift is added together to compute the fluid intake and output for 24 hours. Fluid intake and output is recorded on the nursing intake and output flow sheets. Fluid intake should approximately equal fluid output in a healthy state. If a patient is overhydrated and retaining fluids, she may exhibit edema. In that case, intake has exceeded output. In contrast, if the patient is dehydrated, she has lost fluids, and output has exceeded intake.

19) Intravenous Fluids

Fluids may be given intravenously to replace fluids and electrolytes or to feed patients when gastrointestinal pathology prevents adequate absorption of water or nutrients. Intravenous (IV) lines are also used to administer drugs. A small tube or catheter is inserted directly into a vein, and a tube is attached that leads from the vein to a bag of fluid. The fluid flows out of the bag, through the tube, and into the vein. Nurses may regulate flow rates for IV lines manually by opening or closing a small clamp on the tubing. In many cases, the flow is controlled by an electric pump.

The type and rate of fluid for administration will be found on the Kardex. A special IV therapy record is also kept to document the entire course of IV solutions the patient has received; this record is similar to the medication record. Even if you have not yet learned how to manage an IV, it is important to note on your database that the patient has an IV line, because this is the first step in relating this treatment to the underlying pathology. The presence of an IV means that the patient cannot take fluids, electrolytes, nutrients, or medications orally; otherwise, the IV line would be discontinued.

There are many types of IV fluids used, including dextrose 5% in water (D5W), lactated Ringer's (LR) solution, and normal saline (NS) solution. If you do not recognize the abbreviations used in a patient's medical record, one way to find out exactly what is in the bag is to look at the bag as it hangs near the patient. Once you find out what is in the bag, you can figure out how IV therapy is related to the medical and nursing diagnoses. For example, a dehydrated patient has a fluid volume deficit; therefore, he is receiving dextrose and water to replace fluids.

An IV line is a potential source of infection, because a catheter is going directly into the bloodstream. Therefore, nurses look carefully at where the needle is inserted under the skin and record any signs and symptoms of inflammation, such as redness, swelling, or pain at the site. The dressing over the site must be dry and intact. All of this will be noted on the IV therapy record. The total amount of IV fluids given for the day is also recorded on the nursing flow sheets, under intake for the shift.

20) Elimination

Nurses keep track of elimination very carefully. What goes in has to come out on a regular basis, or else the patient will develop a problem. Elimination includes urine output and bowel movements.

The amount of urine, in milliliters, is recorded on the flow sheet. Any abnormalities in urine color, odor, and quantity will be recorded in the nurse's shift assessment notes, along with pain on elimination or incontinence (loss of control over the bladder, with involuntary urination).

Knowing the patient's urine output is very important. For example, patients who retain fluids have a decreased urine output that could cause or worsen congestive heart failure. Decreased urine output could also indicate renal failure. As you study the pathophysiology of disease, you will recognize how fluid volume deficits and excesses are manifestations of diseases that need to be carefully tracked. Something must be done to treat the patient if the urine output is too high or too low.

Many patients have a special tube to drain urine, called a *urinary catheter*. The tube is usually held in place in the bladder with a balloon. In male patients, it may be held in place externally with a condom-like attachment. The tube leads to a drainage bag. Any patient who has a catheter has an elimination problem, or the tube would not be needed. You need to consider why the catheter is needed, because it relates to the medical and nursing diagnoses. For example, a catheter may be needed in almost anyone who has had surgery of the genitourinary system; watch for bleeding in the urine and keep track of output.

Bowel movements are also very important, because any patient who is immobilized for any reason may be prone to constipation due to decreased peristalsis. Therefore, bowel movements are monitored and recorded on the flow sheets, and any abnormality is documented in the nurses' notes. Check the flow sheet to determine when the patient last had a bowel movement, and check the nurses' notes about problems with constipation, diarrhea, flatus (gas), emesis, or involuntary bowel movements.

Constipation can lead to abdominal discomfort and even impaction, in which the stool creates a blockage and obstructs the bowel. If the bowel is not functioning, the patient may have problems with belching (eructation) or emesis. If gas and solid waste cannot pass downward and out the rectum, they will come out the other end of the gastrointestinal tract as evidenced by belching and emesis.

Postoperatively, patients typically have a decline in bowel functioning because they have been without regular meals. This decline is also related to the decrease in peristalsis that results from immobility and the adverse effects of anesthesia and narcotic pain medications. A healthy sign is the passing of flatus (gas) from the anus: even though the patient has not yet had a bowel movement, one may be impending.

21) Activity

The Kardex will list the patient's activity orders. It is crucial to know what activities the patient can and cannot engage in, to keep her safe from injuries. Carefully assess the patient's ability to walk. The patient's gait may be documented as steady or nonsteady. Note the use of assistive devices such as canes, walkers, or prostheses. The patients may have orders specifying bedrest, chair, and bathroom privileges (BRP); getting up as tolerated; and so on, at the physician's discretion. In hospital settings, patients who are confused or have a decreased level of consciousness may need restraints or side rails elevated on the bed.

In orthopedic patients, knowing the percentage of weight-bearing on the injured bone is essential to preventing falls or further injury to the bone. Typically, weight-bearing is described as a percentage, such as *25% on the right knee* or *50% on the left hip*, or as *toe-touch only*. Abbreviations may be used for activity restrictions such as *no weight-bearing* (NWB) and *weight-bearing as tolerated* (WBAT).

A major concern with activity is ensuring that the patient does not fall; preventing falls is a primary safety issue. Each patient has a fall risk assessment done routinely. This fall risk assessment is a very specific standard of care. Examples of patients that are at high risk for falls include those with decreased levels of consciousness, those with sensory deficits, those receiving pain medications, and those receiving antihypertensive drugs. Review your patient's fall assessment profile and update it to the best of your knowledge based on the data collected. If the risk for falls is great, restraints may be used for safety.

Sleeping is a very important activity. The nurses' notes will indicate whether or not the patient had any problems sleeping. Sleep is an important restorative process and promotes physical healing and cognitive function. Sleep deprivation has many negative consequences, including irritability and increased sensitivity to pain.

Routine Physical Assessment

In inpatient or outpatient settings, you must gather routine head-to-toe physical assessment information at the beginning of the shift or on entry into the outpatient setting. You need to find the most recent physical assessment data available for the patient. Most agencies use a standardized assessment form that contains a checklist with some space for comments. Nurses expand on problem areas in the nurses' notes. When a system to be assessed is within acceptable limits, the nurse may only need to document that by writing *within normal limits* (WNL) or *within designated limits* (WDL). Not writing about normal findings is called *charting by exception,* and saves much time. Documentation is explained in more detail in Chapter 7.

Nurses are required to perform at least one full assessment per shift and check any abnormalities in the assessment much more frequently. As you complete your patient profile database, always record the latest physical assessment data by checking the most recent physical assessment information. The following head-to-toe assessment serves as a review of important information to note on the patient profile database.

22) Vital Signs

Vital signs include blood pressure (BP), temperature (T), pulse (P), and respirations (R). The pain rating is sometimes considered the 5th vital sign. These data provide "vital" information about the key organ systems of the body. The cardiovascular system is assessed with blood pressure and pulse; whereas the lungs are assessed with respirations. Immune functioning, specifically infection, is assessed with body temperature. The pain assessment includes the location, quality, and quantity of pain. The patient's most recent vital signs are typically located on the flow sheets.

23) Height and Weight

Height and weight give an indication of the patient's basic nutritional status. This is found in the nursing admission assessment.

Review of Systems

In a review of systems, which is the major portion of the physical assessment, each system of the body is carefully assessed using the techniques of inspection, palpation, percussion, and auscultation. This information is vital to developing basic nursing diagnoses. Pay close attention to what has been recorded in the most recent nurses' notes and nursing assessments.

24) Neurological and Mental Status

The functioning of the brain is assessed by determining the level of consciousness (LOC) as evidenced by the patient's alertness and orientation to person, place, and time of day. It is important to assess for confusion and disorientation. The patient's speech should be clear and appropriate. The patient's pupils must be equal, round, and reactive to light and accommodation (PERRLA). In addition, the patient should have no deficits in the senses of hearing, vision, taste, or smell. Deficits in any of these areas indicate high *Risk for Injury* as a primary diagnosis. Other nursing diagnoses may include *Bathing, Dressing, Feeding,* or *Toileting Self-Care Deficits, Ineffective Cerebral Tissue Perfusion, Impaired Verbal Communication, Acute* or *Chronic Confusion,* and *Impaired Memory.* The brain controls all motor movements of the body. Motor status is assessed by the patient's ability to move both arms and both legs and to feel sensation, such as pressure and pain, in all limbs. Motor status is recorded with the musculoskeletal system on the patient profile database.

25) Musculoskeletal System

Musculoskeletal problems will be classified under the nursing diagnoses *Activity Intolerance* and *Impaired Physical Mobility.* Deficits in bones, muscles, and joints usually occupy one of the following categories:

- Fracture—any type of break or crack in a bone
- Contracture—tightening and shrinking of muscles from paralysis or fibrosis
- Arthritis—inflammation of a joint
- Spinal curvature—deformed twisting of the bones of the spine

The range of motion (ROM) of each extremity must be recorded under motor abilities. Full range of motion is normal, with decreased range of motion and decreased strength as a result of pathology. Circulation is another important aspect of the musculoskeletal assessment. A circulation check is an assessment of blood flow to the extremities. Most important, circulation checks include distal pulses such as the pedal and tibial pulses in the feet and the radial pulse in the wrist. During the assessment, the nurse observes for pallor, warmth or coolness of the skin, the patient's sense of touch on the injured limb, the amount of edema or swelling in the limb, and the amount of pain reported.

Pulse is the most important source of data about circulation to the limbs. If a pulse is not palpable, a Doppler machine is used to amplify the sound of the pulse in the artery. Lack of a pulse in a limb is a medical emergency; it means that there is no blood circulating to the limb. The tissues will die without oxygen. If the situation is not immediately rectified, it may result in the need to amputate the limb. Pulses in the extremities also indicate the ability of the heart to effectively pump blood to the periphery of the body.

When bones are broken, the patient may need a cast, splint, brace, collar, or other device to immobilize muscles, tendons, or bones. Anyone in a cast needs circulation checks. Sometimes edema causes a cast to become too tight, cutting off circulation in the limb. The cast will need to be removed to restore circulation, or else the patient may have tissue death and the need for amputation of the affected extremity.

Therapeutic treatment devices are often required for improving circulation in the legs. Circulation decreases when the patient is immobilized. With immobility, blood stagnates in the legs, raising the risk of serious complications such as formation of a thrombus, thrombophlebitis, and embolism. A thrombus is a blood clot in a blood vessel; it can irritate and inflame the veins (thrombophlebitis). If the thrombus breaks off from a leg vein and floats freely in the bloodstream, at which point it is called an *embolus,* it can subsequently lodge in a blood vessel in the lung (pulmonary embolism). The reason for treating patients with antiembolic stockings and mechanical sequential compression devices is to improve venous circulation and the return of blood to the heart, thereby preventing the formation of a thrombus.

26) Cardiovascular System

The basic assessment of the heart includes listening to heart sounds and determining whether heart sounds are normal or abnormal, determining whether the heart is beating regularly or irregularly, and assessing for chest pain. The apical pulse rate is assessed at the apical area of the heart, but a thorough assessment includes listening in the aortic, pulmonic, tricuspid, and mitral areas as well. Abnormal heart sounds and rates appear under the nursing diagnoses **Decreased Cardiac Output** and **Risk for Decreased Cardiac Tissue Perfusion.** An indication of congestive heart failure, in which the heart no longer pumps blood effectively, is engorgement of the neck veins, referred to as jugular venous distention (JVD). Chest pain, also known as angina, is a very important symptom that indicates that the heart is not getting enough oxygen. Chest pain needs to be treated immediately, especially in a patient with a chronic or acute condition involving the cardiovascular system.

Assessment of the peripheral vascular system includes assessing all pulses, the same as during the musculoskeletal assessment. Pulses in the limbs are especially important to check, because doing so helps you assess the heart's ability to pump blood to the extremities. If the pulses are not palpable, use the Doppler device to hear them to ensure there is circulation in the limb.

The color of the nail beds and rate of capillary refill in the nails are indications of circulation. The nail beds should be pink. Capillary refill is assessed by depressing a nail bed and releasing it quickly. Depression of the nailtip evacuates the blood and turns the nail bed white. The pink color should return to the nail bed within 3 seconds after you release pressure.

Edema in patients with heart failure usually indicates that a patient is retaining fluid; because the failing heart is not able to pump the blood efficiently and some of the fluid filters into the surrounding tissues. Pitting edema is present when the examiner compresses the edematous area over a bone with the thumb, and a dent remains in the tissue. This indicates excessive fluid in the tissue.

27) Respiratory System

The assessment of the respiratory system includes the depth, rate, and rhythm of breathing, and the use of accessory muscles. Breath sounds are auscultated and are normally clear, without crackles (rales) or wheezes. Cyanosis, or a blue discoloration of the skin or nail beds, indicates a lack of oxygen. A cough may be characterized as productive (producing sputum) or nonproductive (without sputum). When sputum is present, the color and amount are also recorded.

Oxygen therapy is commonly given to treat insufficient oxygenation and the type of therapy will be listed on the Kardex or record. Oxygen is usually given via a nasal cannula (with small tubes extending into the patient's nostrils), a face mask, or a tracheostomy collar. Because oxygen dries out mucous membranes, it is often humidified. Note the flow rate if the patient has oxygen running.

A pulse oximeter is commonly used to evaluate the oxygen saturation of hemoglobin. Record the percentage of oxygen saturation. Note whether the patient has a history of smoking. Nursing diagnoses commonly used for problems in this area include *Impaired Gas Exchange* and *Ineffective Airway Clearance.*

28) Gastrointestinal System

Bowel sounds must be present in all four quadrants of the patient's abdomen. They represent peristalsis, defined as the movement of materials through the gastrointestinal (GI) tract. Bowel sounds in all four quadrants indicate a functional gastrointestinal tract. Absent or decreased bowel sounds may produce a firm, distended abdomen from the accumulation of solid wastes and gas in the bowel. The patient may report abdominal pain and tenderness.

Decreased peristalsis may result in nausea and vomiting.

A common treatment for patients with little or no peristalsis is an NG tube. This tube is inserted into the stomach and attached to suction to remove solids, fluids, and gases until bowel functioning returns to normal. Drainage is carefully measured as part of the patient's output. The color of the output is also described. For example, drainage that is brown or black or resembles coffee grounds may be caused by old dried blood, whereas green indicates bile in the drainage.

Some patients may have an ostomy, which is a surgical opening in the abdominal wall. The intestine is cut and sewn to the opening in the abdomen. If the ostomy involves the colon, the opening is called a colostomy; if it involves the ileum portion of the intestine, it is called an ileostomy. A plastic bag is glued to the abdomen to catch the wastes that would normally be evacuated from the rectum. This surgical procedure is usually done to treat cancer of the bowel when the cancerous portion of the bowel is removed. The color, consistency, and amount of drainage from the ostomy will be recorded in the nurses' notes. In addition, the amount of drainage will be recorded on the flow sheet and tallied in the total patient output for the shift.

29) Skin and Wounds

The skin assessment includes inspection for color and turgor, along with inspection for rashes, bruises, pressure ulcers, surgical wounds, and any other type of wound (such as bullet holes or knife wounds). Describe the size and location of the wound, and whether its edges are approximated. Note if the wound is held together with sutures, staples, Steri-Strips, or other material. A rash may indicate an allergy to a drug or other substance. Bruising may indicate problems with blood clotting. Any type of wound or ulcer must be carefully assessed for infection, and notations must be made in the nurses' notes regarding the progress (or lack of progress) of healing.

When wounds are covered with a dressing, the nurse will note whether the dressing is clean, dry, and intact. Drainage is described for color and quantity. Sometimes a drain is placed inside the wound to facilitate the removal of fluids and promote healing. The drainage tube is connected to a small drainage collection device (container) such as a Jackson-Pratt bulb or a Hemovac drainage system .

Skin assessments also involve checking for possible skin breakdown and development of pressure ulcers, also known as *pressure sores*. The Braden scale or a similar rating form is used to predict a patient's risk of developing a pressure ulcer; it is routinely completed for each patient. Factors predisposing a patient to pressure ulcers include:

▶ Inability to feel pain
▶ Skin that remains moist from perspiration or urine
▶ Lack of activity, such as during bedrest
▶ Lack of mobility or the ability to change body positions
▶ Poor nutrition
▶ The need to be moved up in bed, which can increase the risk of injury from friction and shear

Accreditation standards specify that all patients be assessed for their risk of impaired skin integrity. Find the form used for assessing skin breakdown and update it as needed, based on the most current data you have collected on the patient.

30) Eyes, Ears, Nose, and Throat

The nurse will record data about the patient's eyes, ears, nose, and throat, primarily related to the inspection for signs and symptoms of infection. Infections of these structures are common and bothersome. The signs and symptoms of infection include pain in the form of aching, soreness, or itching, along with redness, drainage, and edema.

Psychosocial and Cultural Assessment

The psychosocial and cultural assessment is very important. The focus of this chapter is on the assessment data that are gathered the night before clinical. Without talking with the patient, only a small amount of data about a patient's psychosocial and cultural background can be collected. The face sheet contains general information

on religious preference, marital status, insurance information, and occupation. Psychosocial and cultural assessments will be further discussed in Chapter 6, which involves mapping of psychosocial problems.

31) Religious Preference

Religion is an important aspect of culture. Many patients practice a religion, such as Judaism, Buddhism, Islam, or Christianity. Of course, there are many variations within and between religious groups. Religious beliefs may influence a patient's view of sickness and the types of treatments that he finds acceptable, and also commonly influence dietary practices and rituals associated with death and dying.

32) Marital Status

Marital status gives one indication of the structure of the patient's family and can be easily obtained the night before clinical. A major function of a healthy family is to be supportive during times of stress. Spouses need to be included in the care plan, because they commonly participate in the care of the patient in the health-care agency and in the home. Determining marital status is one element of the assessment of the patient's social support system.

33) Occupation

Occupation gives an indication of the patient's social status, income, and educational level. During your clinical day with the patient, you will need to further assess whether and when the patient will be able to return to work. By finding out the patient's occupation, you can begin thinking about how the person's ability to work will be affected by her health problems.

34) Health-Care Benefits and Insurance

The type of insurance the patient carries directly influences what medications, treatments, surgeries, and other procedures will and will not be paid for. In addition, insurance may or may not cover extended care or rehabilitation services. Knowing what will be covered by insurance is crucial to the development of the care plan. A key question to think about is whether any community resources are available to help the patient obtain services which he cannot afford to pay for himself.

35) Emotional State

The emotional assessment is very important, so check the nurses' notes for information about the patient's mood. Mood is a reflection of emotions, such as *Anxiety, Hopelessness, Powerlessness,* and *Ineffective Coping.* If you are permitted to meet your patient the day before clinical and introduce yourself, you can make a direct observation of the patient's mood for your records. Does the patient appear happy? Sad? Quiet? Nervous? Write down your impressions on the database.

Obtaining Standardized Forms

Gather all the standardized forms that pertain to your patient. These are printed materials used by the health-care agency with patients that have the same diagnosis as your patient.

Standardized Skin Assessment

The purpose of the standardized skin assessment is to prevent pressure ulcers by estimating the patient's risk of developing them. The risk level is based on mental status, continence, mobility, activity, and nutrition. Those at highest risk have decreased levels of consciousness; incontinence; immobility; bedridden status; and inadequate intake of nutrients. You should know what your patient's risk is for developing an ulcer and plan to prevent this problem. Use the standardized form to estimate your patient's risk of pressure ulcer formation. You will include in your plan of care the prevention of pressure ulcers.

Standardized Falls-Risk Assessment

The purpose of the standardized falls-risk assessment is to prevent injury. Use the standardized fall-risk assessment form to estimate your patient's risk of falling. The risk level is based partly on mental status, with those patients who are confused and disoriented at highest risk. Another risk factor is illness-related debilitation, which causes patients to be light-headed when standing, especially during the first 24 hours postoperatively. Patients with orthostatic hypotension, visual impairments, mobility problems, or an unsteady gait are at risk as well. In addition, many patients take medications, such as sedatives and narcotics that increase their risk of falling. Measures to prevent falls should be incorporated into the nursing plan of care.

Standardized Nursing Care Plans

Many agencies have developed standardized nursing care plans for many common medical diagnoses. The care plans include the typical nursing diagnoses, expected patient outcomes, and associated nursing interventions for a particular health problem.

Clinical Pathways

Clinical pathways (also known as *critical pathways*) are standard care plans that integrate all disciplines involved in a patient's care. This type of care planning has come about because of managed health care. The purpose of a clinical pathway is to coordinate services and decrease costs. Physicians, nurses, physical therapists, nutritionists, and other professionals jointly specify typical day-by-day problems, interventions, and expected outcomes for a specific disease or condition.

Many agencies are in the process of developing clinical pathways, and you may or may not have them to follow. If clinical pathways are being used, make sure you know exactly where your patient is on the pathway for the day you will be providing care. Analyze your patient's progress on the pathway to determine whether she is on time, behind schedule, or ahead of schedule. If she is behind, try to determine the reason for the variation.

Patient Education Materials

Patient education is an important aspect of nursing care. Many agencies have developed patient education materials; others use published booklets. Audiovisual aids may also be available. Take these materials home with you and study them. Integrate them into your plan of care. Be prepared to review educational materials with your patient, as appropriate, during the clinical day.

Communicating With Nursing Staff

Try to get as much patient information as possible on your own, and keep a list of questions about any information you cannot find on your patient. Then discuss that list in detail with your clinical faculty. Many students hesitate to bother nursing staff or other personnel in the agency when they are gathering data to prepare a plan of care. But most busy nurses do not mind answering a few thoughtful questions; after all, they were students once too. Keep in mind, however, that it is your responsibility to gather the relevant data. It is a learning experience for you to search out the information on your own, with clinical supervision from the faculty.

Once you have gathered information from the written records, find the nurse who is responsible for caring for your patient on the day of the assignment. Somewhere in the agency is an assignment sheet that shows all the patient assignments. When you find your patient's nurse, introduce yourself as a student nurse assigned to that patient on the following day. Then ask a very simple open-ended question, such as "Is there anything special I should know about this patient?" Chances are, you will get some good information that may not be written down anywhere. You may even be able to ask one or two more "quick" questions if the nurse has time. Many nurses are glad to have students' help in caring for their patients, and most do not mind answering brief questions if time allows. If the nurse is very busy, she may not have time to talk with you. If so, do not take it personally. The nurses do not know you, and they are busy. Save your remaining questions for your clinical faculty.

CHAPTER 2 SUMMARY

Gathering data is a time-consuming process, at least initially. It gets easier each time you do it, because you become more familiar with where to find the information. The only way you can develop a comprehensive plan of care is to make sure you have complete, accurate assessment data. Sound clinical judgments result from excellent assessments and data analysis.

Your patient profile database comes mainly from your review of patient records. Record keeping in health-care agencies is generally excellent, thanks to standards established by accrediting agencies and the American Nurses Association. In fact, it is required that data about patients be accessible, recorded, and communicated.

The initial patient profile database is focused on pathophysiology and treatments, and has psychological, social, and cultural components. This chapter describes the essential components of the basic patient profile database, the purpose of each component, and the location in the medical records where the information is likely to be found. The patient's current health problems and chronic health problems need to be identified, along with information from a head-to-toe physical assessment. In addition, treatments, medications, IV therapy, laboratory values, and diagnostic tests need to be identified and correlated with the patient's health problems. Diet and activity are also important aspects of treatment, as well as the effects of the health alterations on growth and development, emotional state, and the discomforts typically caused by the patient's health problem.

LEARNING ACTIVITIES

1. Go on a field trip with your clinical group and your clinical faculty to a hospital or outpatient setting. Locate and review the following records: patient charts and information contained in them, such as the face sheet, consent forms, laboratory data, and diagnostic test data; medication records; IV records; the Kardex; nursing flow sheets; nursing assessments; and nurses' notes. Find out where to get the most recent information for each item. For example, perhaps the most recent laboratory data are in the front of the chart. This may vary from agency to agency and even from unit to unit within the agency.

2. After completing the first activity, work alone or with another student to complete a patient profile database with a real patient, using Figure 2.1.

3. As you gather patient data, keep a list of abbreviations that are confusing and need clarification. Usually, each unit has its own set of abbreviations in addition to the standard abbreviations found in most textbooks. Hundreds of abbreviations are used inconsistently and create confusion. For example, DAT may mean *diet as tolerated*, and BKA may mean *below-the-knee amputation*. Write down anything that confuses you, and ask your faculty for clarification. Share your list with others in the clinical group.

4. Find out where the list of patient assignments is posted and track down the staff nurse responsible for your patient. Be assertive, and ask how the patient is doing today. Go into the patient's room and introduce yourself. Ask the patient how he is doing and if you can get him anything. Stay no longer than 5 minutes. If the patient asks for something you cannot do or provide, tell the assigned nurse. Use this exercise to determine what you can assess about your patient's emotional state in just five brief minutes by listening to him and watching his nonverbal behavior.

REFERENCES

1. *Nursing: Scope and Standards of Practice.* 2nd ed. Silver Spring, Md: American Nurses Association; 2010.
2. Erikson EH. *Childhood and Society.* New York, NY: Norton; 1963 (reissued 1993).
3. Schuster PM, Nykolyn L. *Communication for Nurses: How to Prevent Harmful Events and Promote Patient Safety.* Philadelphia, Pa: F.A. Davis; 2010.
4. Tannen D. *You Just Don't Understand: Women and Men in Conversation.* New York, NY: Quill; 2001.
5. Van Leeuwen AM, Poelhuis-Leth, DJ, Bladh, ML. Davis's Comprehensive Handbook of Laboratory and Diagnostic Tests with Nursing Implications. 5th ed. Philadelphia, Pa: F.A. Davis; 2013.

CONCEPT CARE MAPS: GROUPING CLINICAL DATA IN A MEANINGFUL MANNER

OBJECTIVES

1. Identify the American Nurses Association (ANA) standard of professional nursing practice related to analyzing and organizing patient data to determine nursing diagnoses.

2. Identify primary medical diagnoses.

3. Review patient profile data to determine general health problems.

4. Categorize patient profile data according to the patient's response to the health problem.

5. List primary assessments associated with the medical diagnosis.

6. Label nursing diagnoses.

7. Specify relationships between nursing diagnoses.

After gathering patient profile data, the next step in care planning is developing the concept care map. When you finish, the concept care map will contain the primary medical and nursing diagnoses for your patient and all the supporting data (abnormal physical assessment findings, medications, laboratory results, and treatments) categorized and labeled with appropriate nursing diagnoses. In addition, relationships between diagnoses will be identified on the concept care map.

The focus of this chapter is on the second American Nurses Association (ANA) standard of professional nursing practice, which states that the registered nurse analyzes the assessment data to determine the diagnoses or the issues.[1] Concept care maps promote critical analysis of health data in a way that increases the probability of formulating nursing diagnoses accurately. Students are sometimes too quick to put diagnostic labels on patients without data to support the diagnosis, resulting in diagnostic errors.

Concept care maps help students organize data correctly and thus improve the accuracy of the nursing diagnoses.

You will follow three basic steps to develop a concept care map. These steps are based on meaningful learning theory and assimilation theory.[2,3] The first step is to diagram propositions. The second step is to arrange data in hierarchical order. The third step is to make meaningful associations between segments of the diagram. In this chapter, these theoretical steps will be defined with specific examples for application to nursing care plans.

Students are sometimes confused by the words *theory* and *theoretical*. Theories are important because they explain phenomena. Meaningful learning theory and assimilation theory explain how you can increase your critical-thinking abilities by mapping patient care concepts. A concept care map is a useful method for helping nursing students clinically reason and formulate clinical judgments during analysis and organization of patient profile data. Students demonstrate critical thinking when they organize data logically in a concept care map. Critical thinking skills are used during the process of developing patient care maps.

This chapter is intended to give you practice in developing concept care maps for three different patient case studies: a patient with diabetes, a surgical patient with a knee replacement, and a surgical patient with a mastectomy. Patient profile data will be provided for each case study. You will be guided step-by-step in completing a concept care map in the first case study. Case studies 2 and 3 are included in the learning activities at the end of the chapter for additional practice.

Case Study 1: Database for a Patient With Diabetes

Figure 3.1 contains data collected by a student nurse from a patient's records. The patient was hospitalized with newly diagnosed diabetes. The patient profile database is sketchy, but it contains all the information this student collected. Assume that the student has not had much experience in collecting data and that this is her first patient assignment. Carefully review the information in Figure 3.1 to obtain some general ideas

about the patient's problems that will be used for step 1 of concept care mapping. As you review the database, ignore the blank spaces on the form for now. The first step is to formulate initial impressions of the clinical patient profile data.

Step 1. Building a Framework

In step 1, you will diagram the framework of propositions. You must propose or state what you believe to be your patient's key problems based on the data you collected. The key problems are also known as the *concepts*. The framework is the diagram of the key problems, the first step in creating the concept care map. Do this step *before* you start to look up information in your reference materials. The framework of propositions is referred to as the "sloppy copy" version of a concept care map. The objective of doing a sloppy copy is to get the major problems down on a map where you can then critically think and analyze relationships between them. Start by centering the reason for admission to the healthcare setting (often a medical diagnosis) on the sloppy copy of your initial care map. An example of a sloppy copy with the reason for admission is shown in Figure 3.2.

Next, think about the big problems the medical diagnosis has created for this patient, based on the assessment data. He has problems with nutrition and elimination; he is anxious; he has not yet learned how to manage his care at home; and he has an ongoing medical problem of hypertension. Put these problems around the medical diagnosis, like spokes on a wagon wheel, as shown in Figure 3.3.

The next task is to look up information on medical diagnoses, medications, and treatments. The aim of looking up this information is to develop a general understanding of what is wrong with the patient and what is being done by the physician to correct the patient's problems. Assume that you are in your first clinical course, with your first patient assignment, and that you are learning assessment and fundamentals of nursing, including medication administration.

It is now appropriate to attempt to answer some questions about the patient profile data in Figure 3.1. You will need to use course textbooks and software to look up information. Reference materials may include a medical dictionary, a

Student Name: **PMT**

1) Date of Care: **3/23**	2) Patient Initials: **ET**	3) Age: **80** (face sheet)	3) Growth and Development **Ego integrity vs. Despair**	4) Gender: **M** (face sheet)	5) Admission Date: (face sheet) **3/21**

6) Reason for hospitalization (face sheet): Describe reason for hospitalization: (expand on back of page) *Medical Dx:* **Diabetes Type II** *Pathophysiology:* *All signs and symptoms: Highlight those your patient exhibits* **Polydipsia, polyphagia, polyuria, weakness, increased blood glucose, increased glycohemoglobin, glycosuria**	7) Chronic illnesses (physician's history and physical notes in chart; nursing intake assessment and Kardex) **Hypertension**
8) Surgical procedures (consent forms and Kardex): Describe surgical procedure (expand on back of page) Name of surgical procedure: **NA** *Describe surgery:*	

9) ADVANCE DIRECTIVES (NURSE'S ADMISSION ASSESSMENTS):

Living will: ☐ Yes ☐ No	Power of attorney: ☐ Yes ☐ No	Do not resuscitate (DNR) order (Kardex): ☐ Yes ☐ No

10) LABORATORY DATA:

Test	Normal Values	Admission 3/21	Date/Time 3/23	Date/Time	Reason for Abnormal Values
White blood cells (WBCs)					
Red blood cells (RBCs)					
Hemoglobin (Hgb)					
Hematocrit (Hct)					
Platelets					
Prothrombin time (PT)					
International normalized ratio (INR)					
Activated partial thromboplastin time (Aptt)					
Sodium Na					
Potassium K					
Chloride Cl					
Glucose (FBS/BS)		450	120		
Hemoglobin A1C		12%			
Cholesterol		240			
Blood Urea Nitrogen (BUN)					
Creatinine					
Urine analysis (UA)		3+sugar			
Pre-albumin					
Albumin					
Calcium Ca					
Phosphate					
Bilirubin					
Alkaline phosphatase					
SGOT-Serum glutamic-oxyloacetic transaminase					
AST-Serum glutamic pyruvic transaminase					
CK					
CK MB					
Troponin					
B-natriuretic peptide BNP					
pH					
pCO_2					
pO_2					
HCO_3					

11) DIAGNOSTIC TESTS

Chest x-ray:	EKG:	Other abnormal reports:
Sputum or Blood Culture:	Other:	Other:

● Figure 3.1 Patient profile database. Case Study 1: Patient newly diagnosed with diabetes.

12) MEDICATIONS

List medications and times of administration (medication administration record and check the drawer in the carts for spelling). Include over-the-counter (OTC) products/herbal medicines.

		qam 0730	qam 0900	q4h pm	
Times Due					
Brand Name		**Humulin N**	**Diovan**	**Tylenol**	
Generic Name		**NPH Insulin**	**Valsartan**	**Acetaminophen**	
Dose		**35U**	**80mg**	**650mg**	
Administration Route					
Classification					
Action					
Reason This Patient is Receiving					
Pharmacokinetics		O P D 1/2 M E	O P D 1/2 M E	O P D 1/2 M E	O P D 1/2 M E
Contraindications					
Major Adverse Side Effects					
Nursing Implications					
Pt/Family Teaching					

Developed by P. Testa, YSU

ALLERGIES/PAINS

13) Allergies: Type of Reaction: (medication administration record):	14) When was the last time pain medication given? (medication administration record)
14) Where is the pain? (nurse's notes)	14) How much pain is the patient in on a scale 0-10? (nurse's notes, flow sheet):

TREATMENTS

15) List treatments (Kardex): Rationale for treatments:

Glucometer qid ac & hs
VS q4h
Position changes q2h
Ted hose
IS q1h while awake
C&DB q1h while awake

16) Support services (Kardex) What do support services provide for the patient? **Dietitian and Diabetes Educator**

17) What does the consultant do for the patient?:

18) DIET/FLUIDS

Type of Diet (Kardex): **1800 ADA**	Restrictions (Kardex): **No sugar added**	Gag reflex intact: [X] Yes ☐ No	Appetite: [X] Good ☐ Fair ☐ Poor	Breakfast **100** %	Lunch **100** %	Dinner **100** %

What type of diet is this?:

What types of foods are included in this diet and what foods should be avoided?:

Circle Those Problems That Apply:

Prior 24 hours Fluid intake: (Oral & IV) **2200** Fluid output **1800** (flow sheet)	• Problems: swallowing, chewing, dentures (nurse's notes) • Needs assistance with feeding (nurse's notes) • Nausea or vomiting (nurse's notes) • Overhydrated or dehydrated (evaluate total intake and output on flow sheet
Tube feedings: Type and rate (Kardex)	• Belching: • Other:_____

19) INTRAVENOUS FLUIDS (IV therapy record)

Type and Rate: **NA**	IV dressing dry, no edema, redness of site: ☐ Yes ☐ No	Other:

20) ELIMINATION (flow sheet)

Last bowel movement:	Foley/condom catheter: ☐ Yes ☐ No
Circle Those Problems That Apply:	

- Bowel: constipation, diarrhea, flatus, incontinence, belching
- Urinary: hesitancy, frequency, burning, incontinence, odor
- Other: _____
- What is causing the problem in elimination? **History of polyuria**

21) ACTIVITY (Kardex, flow sheet)

Ability to walk (gait): **Unsteady**	Type of activity orders: **OOB/chair**	Use of assistance devices: cane, walker, crutches, prosthesis:	Falls-risk assessment rating:
No. of side rails required (flow sheet) **2**	Restraints (flow sheet): ☐ Yes ☒ No	Weakness ☒ Yes ☐ No	Trouble sleeping (nurse's notes): ☐ Yes ☐ No

What does activity order mean?: _____
Why isn't the patient up ad lib?: _____
Would the problem cause weakness?: _____

PHYSICAL ASSESSMENT DATA

22) BP (flow sheet): **132/92**	2) TPR (flow sheet): **98.4-77-18**	23) Height: **5' 10"** Weight: **174** (nursing intake assessments)

24) NEUROLOGICAL/MENTAL STATUS:

LOC: alert and oriented to person, place, time (A&O x 3), confused, etc. **A&Ox3**	Speech: clear, appropriate/inappropriate **Clear**
Pupils: PERRLA **PERRLA**	Sensory deficits for vision/hearing/taste/ smell **Glasses**

25) MUSCULOSKELETAL STATUS:

Bones, joints, muscles (fractures, contractures, arthritis, spinal curvatures, etc):	Extremity (temperature, edema (pitting vs. nonpitting) & sensation)
Motor: ROM x 4 extremities **Full ROM**	
Ted hose/plexi pulses/compression devices: type:	Casts, splint, collar, brace:

26) CARDIOVASCULAR SYSTEM:

Pulses (radial, pedal) (to touch or with Doppler): **3+ pedals & radials**	Capillary refill (<3s): ☐ Yes ☐ No	
Neck vein (distention):	Sounds: S1, S2, regular, irregular: Apical rate: **76 rrr**	Any chest pain:

27) RESPIRATORY SYSTEM:

Depth, rate, rhythm: **20**	Use of accessory muscles:	Cyanosis:	Sputum color, amount:	Cough: productive nonproductive	Breath sounds: clear, rales, wheezes **Clear**
Use of oxygen: nasal cannula, mask, trach collar:	Flow rate of oxygen:	Oxygen humidification: ☐ Yes ☐ No		Pulse oximeter: _____ % oxygen saturation	Smoking: ☐ Yes ☐ No

28) GASTROINTESTINAL SYSTEM

Abdominal pain, tenderness, guarding; distention, soft, firm: **Soft, nondistended**	Bowel sounds x 4 quadrants: **Present 4 quads**	NG tube: describe drainage
Ostomy: describe stoma site and stools:	Other:	

● Figure 3.1 Continued

29) SKIN AND WOUNDS:

Color, turgor: **Pink**	Rash, bruises:	Describe wounds (size, locations):	Edges approximated: ☐ Yes ☐ No	Type of wound drains:
Characteristics of drainage:	Dressings (clean, dry, intact):	Sutures, staples, steri-strips, other:	Risk for pressure ulcer assessment rating:	Other:

30) EYES, EARS, NOSE, THROAT (EENT):

Eyes: redness, drainage, edema, ptosis	Ears: drainage	Nose: redness, drainage, edema	Throat: sore
Psychosocial and Cultural Assessment			
31) Religious preference (face sheet) **Catholic**	32) Marital status (face sheet) **Widower**	33) Health care benefits and insurance (face sheet): **Blue Cross/Blue Shield**	
34) Occupation (face sheet) **Retired**	35) Emotional state (nurse's notes) **Anxious about giving insulin and following diet**		

● Figure 3.1 Continued

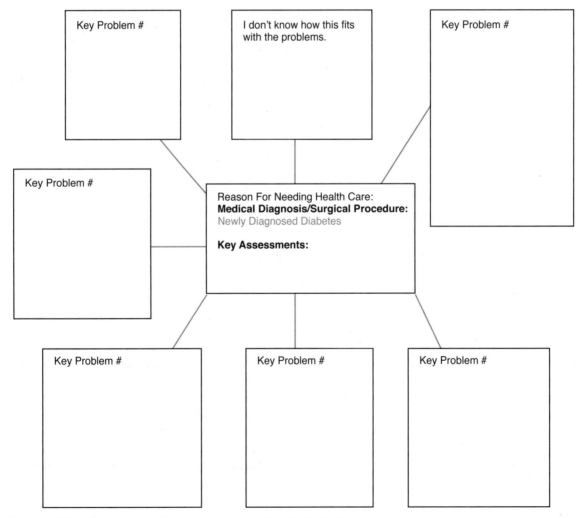

● Figure 3.2   Sloppy copy with reason for admission highlighted.

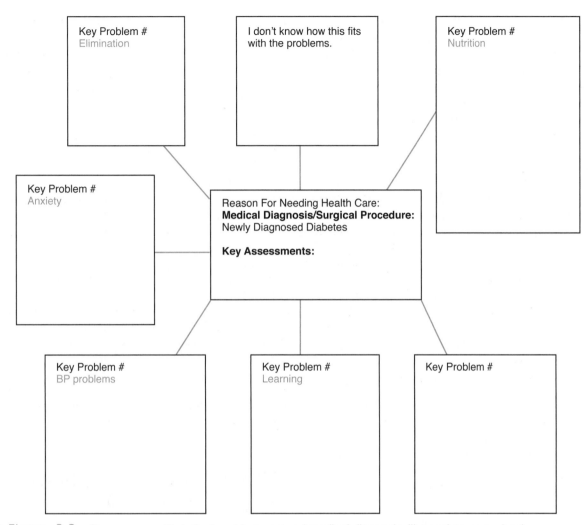

● Figure 3.3   Sloppy copy with patient problems around medical diagnosis, like spokes on a wheel.

manual of laboratory and diagnostic procedures, a book on nutrition therapy, a drug handbook or pharmacology book, a standardized care plan book, a fundamentals textbook, and a medical-surgical textbook. You may use software programs and Internet sites, which decrease the amount of time required to research materials, such as computerized drug guides[4] or computerized nursing care plans.[5] There is also an Internet site called Ask.com (www.ask.com) that provides information about many topics. Go to the site, ask a question, and you will get an answer. For example, ask for patient education material about diabetes and you will find all kinds of information in an instant. Be careful that the information you retain is from a reliable source and the information is based on research.

Looking Up Information

For this patient, you will need to look up information about drugs, laboratory and diagnostic tests, diet, and medical diagnoses.

Drugs

Start by looking up drugs. There are only three for this patient: Humulin N (NPH insulin), Diovan (valsartan), and Tylenol (acetaminophen). You may be thinking, "Why start with drugs?" Medication administration is one of the most dangerous things nurses do, and it is a primary focus of fundamentals courses. Therefore, before you use your energy looking up everything else, invest some time when your mind is fresh, reading and taking some notes on the drugs. Patient education with regard to drugs is a key nursing responsibility. Determine the type of information that the patient needs to know about taking his drugs properly at home.

Laboratory and Diagnostic Tests

Next, read about the laboratory and diagnostic tests in a laboratory and diagnostic procedures manual. Medication administration is often based on laboratory values. There is a direct relationship between laboratory values and the patient's medication. You must identify those relationships. Make sure you know the most up-to-date laboratory values before you administer drugs. Also, patient teaching is needed regarding laboratory tests, so you must identify what the patient needs to know about the diagnostic tests that have been ordered.

Diet

Obtain information on the patient's prescribed diet. How is the diet related to the medical diagnosis? What patient education is needed regarding diet? What is a sample menu for the patient? If you have a nutritional therapy book, at least one chapter will be devoted to diabetes. If you do not have a nutrition book, this would be a good topic on which to try the *www.ask.com* Web site. Ask for information about diabetic diets.

Medical Diagnoses/Chronic Illnesses

Find information about the patient's medical diagnoses. Your fundamentals text may not offer much help because many fundamentals books contain little disease-specific information. The aim of a fundamentals text is to teach the foundational skills essential to providing care for basic human needs. Fundamentals courses typically do not cover specific aspects of medical-surgical nursing care. Therefore, you may find a medical dictionary helpful to briefly define the disease and provide a concise description of symptoms, etiology, complications, treatments, prognosis, and nursing implications.

The most detailed information about diseases can be found in a medical-surgical nursing text. In fact, it is a good investment to buy a medical-surgical text ahead of time, so that you can use the book as a reference in your fundamentals course. You may find certain Web sites helpful as well, such as those shown in Box 3.1.

Other helpful references include standardized care plan guidelines and clinical pathways. These may be obtained from the health-care agency or from standardized care planning manuals.[5] Standardized care plans include patient goals, patient outcomes, nursing interventions, and rationales. Clinical pathways also integrate the services of other health professionals in attaining patient goals. These are general guidelines, not specific to a particular patient. The concept care map that you develop will be specific to your patient on the day you provide care for him.

As you review standardized plans and pathways, you must sort through all the possible nursing diagnoses, goals, objectives, and interventions; then you must determine what is appropriate for the day you are assigned to care for the patient. This has been called *individualizing* the plan of care. This is difficult at first, but with practice and experience, you will get better at it. An important

---

Box 3.1   WEB SITES: GATHERING INFORMATION

American Heart Association
    www.heart.org
Arthritis Foundation www.arthritis.org
National Cancer Institute
    www.cancer.gov
American Diabetes Association
    www.diabetes.org
Immunization Action Coalition
    www.immunize.org
American Lung Association
    www.lung.org
Internet Mental Health
    www.mentalhealth.com
National Kidney Foundation
    www.kidney.org
National Institute of Neurological Disorders
    and Stroke www.ninds.nih.gov

point to remember as you review information from standardized plans is that you must determine what is most relevant to the patient at the point in time you are assigned to care for him.

Preventing Falls and Skin Breakdown

The next step in building a concept care map for your diabetic patient is to analyze his risk for falls and skin breakdown. Preventing falls and skin breakdown is fundamental to competent nursing care. Accrediting agencies require that all patients be evaluated for falls and skin breakdown; thus, each agency will have assessment forms for this task. Sample assessment forms, with data from this case study, are shown in Figures 3.4 and 3.5. These have been filled out based on patient profile data and on general knowledge about patients with diabetes. Thus, the specifics of the data collected and general information for a patient with diabetes are used to complete the assessments. You must rate your patient for falls and skin breakdown based on the most current information you have obtained on the patient.

When assessing the patient's risk of falling, as shown in Figure 3.4, consider that the patient is over age 60, he is weak, he has had problems with urinary frequency, and he is taking an antihypertensive.[6] By looking up information, you may conclude that his weakness is from inadequate nutrition and dehydration. Urinary frequency is associated with polyuria; the antihypertensive drug may contribute to orthostatic hypotension; and decreased muscle tone and strength may be associated with aging. Therefore, this patient is at **Risk for Falls.** Write the fall risk score and your clinical judgment that the patient is at risk for falls in the upper right box of the assessment form.

Next, assess the patient's risk for development of pressure ulcers. Each patient is assessed for potential problems in development of skin breakdown. This skin breakdown is termed a *pressure ulcer* or *pressure sore*. Figure 3.5 shows the Braden Scale for Predicting Pressure Ulcer Risk.[7] To assess a patient's risk, score the patient on each of the six subscales and total the points. The maximum score is 23, which indicates little or no risk. A score between 10 and 16 indicates a risk of pressure ulcers. A score of 9 or less indicates a high risk of pressure ulcers.

How would you rate the diabetic patient in this scenario? Based on data from the patient's profile, the patient does not have any sensory impairments (4 points); is probably rarely moist (4 points); probably walks occasionally (3 points); probably has slightly limited mobility from being only out of bed and in a chair (OOB/chair) (3 points); has excellent nutrition (4 points); and has a potential problem with friction and shear (2 points). He has 20 of 23 points based on the evidence provided in the patient profile database. Thus, he has a low risk for developing a pressure ulcer. Write the total pressure ulcer risk score in the box in the lower right corner of the assessment form and then also write your clinical judgment that the patient is at low risk for developing a pressure ulcer in this box.

There are many assessments that you may need to do, depending on the course you are taking and the condition of the patient. For example, there is an assessment for pain shown in Figure 3.6 and an assessment for neurological functioning shown in Figure 3.7.

At this point, you have completed the patient profile database and looked up basic information about the disease and its treatment. It is now time to categorize the data you have gathered under the basic problems you identified on your map. All the pieces of data must be organized into a hierarchical and comprehensive pattern.

Step 2: Mapping the Hierarchy

According to educational theory, concept maps are hierarchical graphical organizers. A hierarchy is a series of consecutive classes or groups. For example, one hierarchy in biology is the classification of living things into kingdom, phylum, class, order, family, genus, and species. Subconcepts are organized in a pattern under major concepts, to facilitate understanding of relationships and to organize information. The graph of the hierarchy is a picture or map of the organized relationships between concepts and subconcepts.

In concept care mapping, the subconcepts are the specific pieces of data that were collected about the patient and support the major problems

RISK FOR FALLS
ASSESSMENT

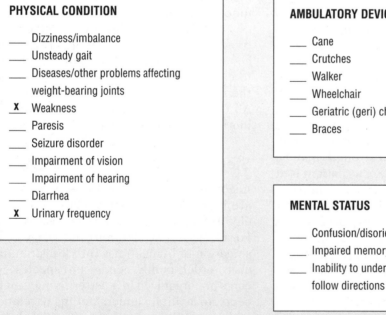

DIRECTIONS: Place an "x" in front of elements that apply to your patient. Based on the assessment, check whatever applies to the patient. A patient for whom you place four or more "x" marks is at risk for falling

Total Score ___4___   Clinical Judgment

At risk for Falling

GENERAL DATA

X Age over 60
___ History of falls before admission
___ Postoperative/admitted for operation
___ Smoker

MEDICATIONS

___ Diuretics or diuretic effects
X Hypotensive or CNS suppressant drugs
___ Postoperative/admitted for operation
(e.g., narcotic, sedative, psychotropic, hypnotic, tranquilizer, antihypertensive, antidepressant)
___ Medication that increases GI motility

PHYSICAL CONDITION

___ Dizziness/imbalance
___ Unsteady gait
___ Diseases/other problems affecting weight-bearing joints
X Weakness
___ Paresis
___ Seizure disorder
___ Impairment of vision
___ Impairment of hearing
___ Diarrhea
X Urinary frequency

AMBULATORY DEVICES USED

___ Cane
___ Crutches
___ Walker
___ Wheelchair
___ Geriatric (geri) chair
___ Braces

MENTAL STATUS

___ Confusion/disorientation
___ Impaired memory or judgment
___ Inability to understand or follow directions

● Figure 3.4   Assessing risk for falls. Perform this assessment before the clinical day. (From Brians LK, et al. The development of the RISK tool for fall prevention. *Rehabilitation Nursing*. 1991;16[2]:67, with permission.)

Directions: Add up the total points, a perfect score is 23. A high score means lower risk for pressure ulcer. A low score means higher risk for pressure ulcer.

BRADEN SCALE >>> *FOR PREDICTING PRESSURE SORE RISK*

| Patient's Name: | | Evaluator's Name: | | Date of Assessment: | |

	1	2	3	4
SENSORY PERCEPTION Ability to respond meaningfully to pressure-related discomfort	Completely limited: Unresponsive (does not moan, flinch, or grasp) to painful stimuli, due to diminished level of consciousness or sedation, OR limited ability to feel pain over most of the body surface.	Very Limited: Responds only to painful stimuli. Cannot communicate discomfort except by moaning or restlessness, OR has a sensory impairment which limits the ability to feel pain or discomfort over 1/2 of the body.	Slightly Limited: Responds to verbal commands but cannot always communicate discomfort or need to be turned, OR has a sensory impairment which limits ability to feel pain or discomfort in 1 or 2 extremities.	No Impairment: Responds to verbal commands. Has no sensory deficit which would limit ability to feel or voice pain or discomfort.
MOISTURE Degree to which skin is exposed to moisture	Constantly Moist: Skin is kept moist almost constantly by perspiration, urine, etc. Dampness is detected every time patient is moved or turned.	Moist: Skin is often but not always moist. Linen must be changed at least once a shift.	Occasionally Moist: Skin is occasionally moist, requiring an extra linen change approximately once a day.	Rarely Moist: Skin is usually dry; linen requires changing only at routine intervals.
ACTIVITY Degree of physical activity	Bedfast: Confined to bed.	Chairfast: Ability to walk severely limited or nonexistent. Cannot bear own weight and/or must be assisted into chair or wheelchair.	Walks Occasionally: Walks occasionally during day but for very short distances, with or without assistance. Spends majority of each shift in bed or chair.	Walks Frequently: Walks outside the room at least twice a day and inside room at least once every 2 hours during walking hours.
MOBILITY Ability to change and control body position	Completely Immobile: Does not make even slight changes in body or extremity position without assistance.	Very Limited: Makes occasional slight changes in body or extremity position but unable to make frequent or significant changes independently.	Slightly Limited: Makes frequent though slight changes in body or extremity position independently.	No Limitations: Makes major and frequent changes in position without assistance.
NUTRITION Usual food intake pattern	Very Poor: Never eats a complete meal. Rarely eats more than 1/3 of any food offered. Eats 2 servings or less of protein (meat or dairy products) per day. Takes fluids poorly. Does not take a liquid dietary supplement, OR is NPO and/or maintained on clear liquids or IVs for more than 5 days.	Probably Inadequate: Rarely eats a complete meal and generally eats only about 1/2 of any food offered. Protein intake includes 3 servings of meat or dairy products per day. Occasionally will take a dietary supplement, OR receives less than optimum amount of liquid diet or tube feeding.	Adequate: Eats over half of meals. Eats a total of 4 servings of protein (meat, dairy products) each day. Occasionally will refuse a meal, but will usually take a supplement if offered, OR is on a tube feeding or TPN regimen, which probably meets most of nutritional needs.	Excellent: Eats most of every meal. Never refuses a meal. Usually eats a total of 4 or more servings of meat and dairy products. Occasionally eats between meals. Does not require supplementation.
FRICTION AND SHEAR	Problem: Requires moderate to maximum assistance in moving. Complete lifting without sliding against sheets is impossible. Frequently slides down in bed or chair, requiring frequent repositioning with maximum assistance. Spasticity, contractures, or agitation leads to almost constant friction.	Potential Problem: Moves feebly or requires minimum assistance. During a move skin probably slides to some extent against the sheets, chair, restraints, or other devices. Maintains relatively good position in chair or bed most of the time but occasionally slides down.	No Apparent Problem: Moves in bed and in chair independently and has sufficient muscle strength to lift up completely during move. Maintains good position in bed or chair at all times.	Total Points: _____ Clinical Judgment _____ _____ _____ _____

● Figure 3.5   Braden Scale for Predicting Pressure Ulcer Assessment. (From Braden B, Bergstrom, N. In: Bryant RA, ed. *Acute and Chronic Wounds: Nursing Management*. St. Louis, Mo: Mosby; 1992.)

Initial Pain Assessment Tool

Patient's Name _____ Date _____

Diagnosis _____ Age _____ Room _____

Physician _____

Nurse _____

1. LOCATION: Patient or nurse mark drawing.

2. INTENSITY: Patient rates the pain. Scale used _____
    Present: _____
    Worst pain gets: _____
    Best pain gets: _____
    Acceptable level of pain: _____

3. QUALITY: (Use patient's own words, e.g., prick, ache, burn, throb, pull, sharp) _____
    _____

4. ONSET, DURATION, VARIATIONS, RHYTHMS: _____

5. MANNER OF EXPRESSING PAIN: _____
    _____
    _____

6. WHAT RELIEVES THE PAIN? _____
    _____
    _____

7. WHAT CAUSES OR INCREASES THE PAIN? _____
    _____
    _____

8. EFFECTS OF PAIN: (Note decreased function, decreased quality of life.)
    Accompanying symptoms (e.g., nausea) _____
    Sleep _____
    Appetite _____
    Physical activity _____
    Relationship with others (e.g., irritability) _____
    Emotions (e.g., anger, suicidal, crying) _____
    Concentration _____
    Other _____

9. OTHER COMMENTS: _____
    _____

10. PLAN: _____
    _____
    _____

● Figure 3.6   Initial pain assessment tool, for use during the clinical day. (From DeLaune S, Ladner P. *Fundamentals of Nursing: Standards and Practice*. Albany, NY: Delmar Thomson Learning; 2002.)

Clinical Judgment_____

you identified on the spokes of the wheel surrounding the reason for admission to the healthcare setting. The subconcepts that must be classified are the clinical pathological signs and symptoms the patient displayed, treatments, medications, laboratory data, and chronic illness data. You must sift through the data once more and categorize them.

Keep in mind that a concept care map is based on actual problems. Consequently, you should categorize only abnormal patient data. This is one reason why it is important for you to look up information on the patient's disease, drugs, treatments, surgery, and so on before categorizing the data; that way, you have general knowledge of the main treatments for the primary medical diagnosis and surgical procedures.

The problems that extend out from the central reason for admission will become nursing diagnoses based on the definitions and classifications of the North American Nursing Diagnosis Association (NANDA).[8] Categorize all the data you have *before* assigning any diagnostic labels.

Start by reviewing the physical assessment data; try categorizing abnormal data in appropriate boxes. If an item belongs in more than one box, put it in two or more places. If you do not know where an item goes, place it in the central box labeled "I don't know how this fits with the problems," as shown in Figure 3.8. This is a

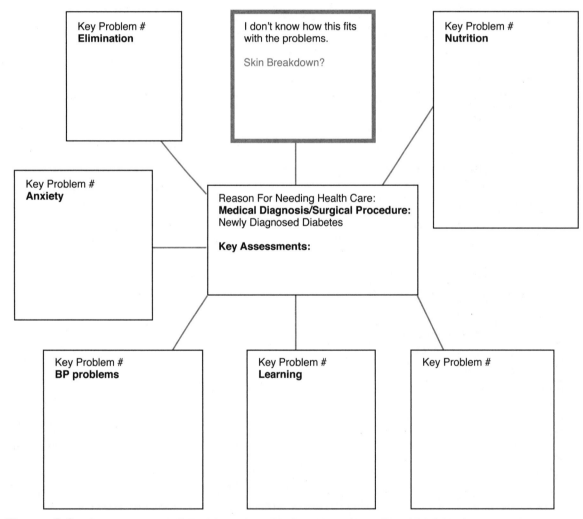

● Figure 3.8   Sloppy copy with "I don't know how this fits with problems" box highlighted.

very important box. There are times when you may find medications the patient should not be taking, or treatments the patient should not be receiving and that need to be discontinued.

Now try to add remaining pieces of abnormal data into the boxes. For example, add information about drugs (Humulin N, Diovan, Tylenol), laboratory test results (serum glucose 450 down to 120, glycosylated hemoglobin = 12%, cholesterol 40, urine 3+ sugar), treatments (glucometer [Accu-Chek, VS qid), diet (1800 American Diabetes Association [ADA], no added sugar), activity (OOB/chair, risk of falls), and psychosocial cultural data (anxiety about injections and diet, widower). Now your map might look like Figure 3.9.

You must be able to explain why you put each item in the box you selected. Be prepared to explain how abnormal physical assessment findings are related to pathophysiology and the need for specific diagnostic tests, medications, and treatments. You must demonstrate knowledge of the pathophysiology, diagnosis, and treatment of the patient's disease.

A number of items are listed at the top of the map in the box labeled "I don't know how this fits with the problems," items that do not seem to fit in any of the other boxes. If you look at these items as a group, they suggest that the patient is not as mobile as he should be and that he has a risk of falling. This realization warrants adding

● Figure 3.9 Sloppy copy with abnormal data added to boxes.

another box to your map to address the patient's mobility problem. The symptom of weakness also goes along with this problem of mobility. Therefore, a key problem is immobility; and this problem is placed in a separate box, as in Figure 3.10.

Suppose you are still not sure about the remaining items in the "I don't know how this fits with the problems" box: acetaminophen, widower, and skin breakdown. This means you have not collected enough data to make decisions about those items, and you need to do more assessment when you meet with the patient the next day. For example, you need to find out whether the acetaminophen was prophylactic and never used. Did the patient have pain somewhere? Was he running a temperature?

What type of social support does the patient have as a widower? The answer to this question could have major implications if he has no one at home to help him accomplish the self-care tasks he cannot complete on his own. He may need nursing home placement or home health care.

What about the skin breakdown? The patient does not have any specific problems noted in the data, but from your reading you may have noted that diabetics have trouble with circulation and sensation in their legs and feet, making them prone to skin breakdown. In addition, their wounds heal slowly. The patient needs to be taught foot care and methods to prevent skin breakdown.

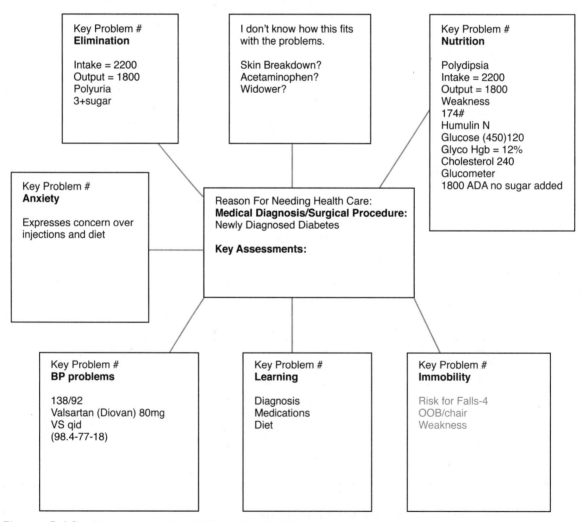

● Figure 3.10   Sloppy copy with mobility problem highlighted.

Adding Assessments for Primary Medical Diagnoses

Now that you have most of your patient data arranged on your concept care map, you should add key assessments to the central box that contains the reason (the medical diagnosis) for admission to the health-care setting. These are important assessments that you will focus on while you are with the patient. The results of these assessments will tell you whether the patient is making progress toward a healthier state in which his diabetes is under control.

In a patient with diabetes, the key assessments consist of watching for hypoglycemia or hyperglycemia and assessing blood glucose levels. Hypoglycemia typically causes weakness, dizziness, sluggishness, hunger, irritability, sweating, paleness, a rapid heart rate, tremors, headache, and changes in mental functioning, such as confusion. The potential for hypoglycemia in the hospital setting is high until food intake, exercise, and the amount of insulin the patient receives are in careful balance. The classic signs of hyperglycemia and ketosis are polydipsia (excessive thirst), polyuria (excessive urination), and polyphagia (excessive appetite). The most important problem to watch for in this patient is an insulin reaction. When giving the patient his insulin, make sure you know his blood glucose level and that he is going to eat if you are giving a dose before eating a meal. Always monitor vital signs. The center of the care map should look like Figure 3-11.

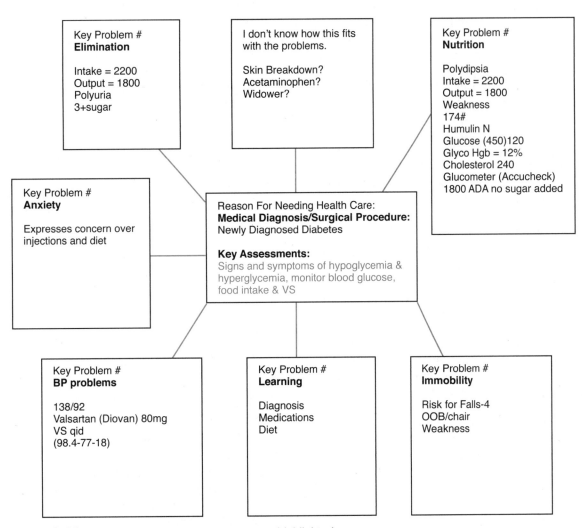

● Figure 3.11   Sloppy copy with key assessments highlighted.

Labeling Nursing Diagnoses

Remember to attach nursing diagnoses labels to problems *after* carefully considering all of the data. Many students have a tendency to select nursing diagnoses too quickly, without first looking at and organizing the data. The net result of making quick decisions about diagnoses is that the diagnoses are often wrong. Therefore, take time to look at the data before you leap into the diagnoses.

Assigning correct diagnoses is essential to developing an individualized plan of care that includes appropriate goals, outcomes, objectives, and interventions specific to the day you are assigned to care for the patient. It will be impossible to develop an individualized plan if you have not accurately identified and prioritized the patient's specific problems. Once you have done so, it is relatively easy to find information on what to do to correct those problems. Developing the plan of care once the correct diagnoses are made is the subject of Chapter 4.

Nursing diagnoses are statements that describe the patient's actual or potential responses to health problems or life processes that the nurse is licensed and competent to treat.[8-13] Nursing diagnoses are focused on the patient's responses to a health problem. In contrast, medical diagnoses are focused on the health problem itself, based on the signs and symptoms related to the pathophysiology of the disease. Medical and nursing diagnoses are inextricably linked, and you, as the nurse, must recognize the linkages. The linkages between the medical and nursing diagnoses are clearly shown by the lines between the medical and nursing diagnoses on the concept care map. The nursing diagnoses flow outward from the primary medical diagnosis like spokes on a wheel. You will continue to grow in your knowledge of nursing diagnoses and medical diagnoses with each day of clinical experience.

For the medical diagnosis of diabetes, the resulting general problems that you identified are elimination, nutrition, learning, anxiety, blood pressure problems, and immobility. These are actual, not potential, problems and you have evidence to substantiate each of them. There are many potential problems in any patient care situation, but the concept care map is focused on actual problems.

The nursing diagnoses have been placed into frameworks that group them in categories and make them easier to locate. Nursing diagnoses have been arranged according to Maslow's[12] hierarchy of needs:

- Physiological needs
- Safety and security
- Love and belonging
- Self-esteem
- Self-actualization

They have also been organized according to Gordon's[13] Functional Health Patterns, which include:

- Health perception/health management
- Nutritional-metabolic pattern
- Elimination pattern
- Activity-exercise pattern
- Sleep-rest pattern
- Cognitive-perceptual pattern
- Self-perception–self-concept pattern
- Role-relationship pattern
- Sexuality-reproductive pattern
- Coping-stress tolerance pattern
- Value-belief pattern

Doenges and Moorhouse's Diagnostic Divisions framework of nursing diagnoses includes:

- Activity/Rest
- Circulation
- Ego Integrity
- Elimination
- Food/Fluid
- Hygiene
- Neurosensory
- Pain/Discomfort
- Respiration
- Safety
- Sexuality
- Social Interaction
- Teaching/Learning

A fourth framework is NANDA's[8] Domains of Nursing Diagnoses:

- Heath Promotion
- Nutrition
- Elimination and Exchange
- Activity/Rest
- Perception/Cognition
- Self-Perception

▶ Role Relationships
▶ Sexuality
▶ Coping/Stress Tolerance
▶ Life Principles
▶ Safety/Protection
▶ Comfort
▶ Growth/Development

Each nursing diagnosis you select for your map must be based on an accurate assessment of the patient's problems.

Each of the problem areas identified for the diabetic patient in the case study will be described, with an explanation of the critical thinking that was needed to determine the final nursing diagnosis for each problem.

Elimination

The data we have to support the problem is the patient's polyuria, which is a classic symptom of hyperglycemia. In addition, the patient is spilling glucose into his urine, also a classic sign of hyperglycemia. The patient's output is currently less than his input, which is likely to be a compensatory response by the body to the dehydrated state caused by polyuria. A review of the list of nursing diagnoses indicates that the diagnosis of *Impaired Urinary Elimination* is probably correct. To confirm the diagnosis, look up its definition, which says, "dysfunction in urine elimination."[8] This fits well with the data you have collected.

Nutrition

A patient with diabetes definitely has nutritional problems. This patient is on the 1800-calorie diabetic diet with no added sugar and is receiving insulin to regulate his blood glucose. A glucometer is being used regularly to monitor his blood glucose level, and his glycosylated hemoglobin is elevated. In addition, the patient's cholesterol is elevated, a problem that should be controlled to decrease his risk of coronary artery disease. The patient's records indicate that he had polydipsia and that his intake currently exceeds his output, probably to compensate for the dehydration that occurred before his blood glucose was regulated with replacement of insulin. The weakness is related to the starvation and dehydration that occurred without adequate insulin. Although the patient appears to be getting better, the diagnosis of *Imbalanced Nutrition: Less Than Body Requirements* is appropriate. It is defined as "intake of nutrients insufficient to meet metabolic needs."[8]

Learning

All patients newly diagnosed with any disease need to learn about self-care. In this case, the patient needs to learn about the disease and prevention of complications. This includes learning about medications, the 1800 ADA diet, care of the feet, and exercise. Foot care and exercise should be added to the box that addresses the patient's learning needs. The appropriate diagnosis is *Deficient Knowledge,* defined as "absence or deficiency of cognitive information related to a specific topic."[8]

Anxiety

The patient said that he is anxious about learning to give himself injections and about following his diet. The diagnosis of *Anxiety* is defined as "a vague uneasy feeling of discomfort or dread accompanied by an autonomic response; the source is often nonspecific or unknown to the individual; a feeling of apprehension caused by anticipation of danger. It is an alerting signal that warns of impending danger and enables the individual to take measures to deal with threat."[8] At this point, the patient appears to be a little anxious, probably because he does not know what is involved or whether he will be capable of caring for himself.

Blood Pressure Problems

The patient is receiving a blood pressure medication and has a slightly elevated diastolic blood pressure. Diabetes affects blood vessels all over the body, and most diabetics eventually develop cardiovascular and peripheral vascular disease. An appropriate nursing diagnosis is *Ineffective Peripheral Tissue Perfusion,* defined as "decrease in blood circulation to the periphery that may compromise health."[8] The patient will need instruction on slowing down the development of peripheral vascular complications, although these complications are inevitable. Peripheral vascular complications of diabetes will affect circulation and sensation in the extremities, with skin breakdown and ulcerations as common consequences. Also, with diabetes, healing of wounds is much slower than normal. It is clear now that the skin breakdown risk that you put in the box labeled "I don't know how this fits with the problems" at the top of the map fits well with *Ineffective Peripheral Tissue Perfusion.*

Mobility

The patient has an increased risk of falling caused by weakness, and he is permitted to be OOB/chair. He can be diagnosed with *Impaired Physical*

Mobility, which is defined as a "limitation in independent, purposeful physical movement of the body or of one or more extremities."[8] Your map should now look like Figure 3.12.

Step 3: Mapping Cross-Links

Your concept care map is almost complete. Step 3 involves analyzing the relationships between the nursing diagnoses in order to make meaningful associations. The links must be accurate, meaningful, and complete. In concept care maps, the concepts you must link are the nursing diagnoses.

You must be able to state explicitly why you believe the diagnoses are related. Your faculty will be able to look at your map and see what was

● Figure 3.12   Sloppy copy with NANDA labels highlighted.

(or was not) in your mind and ask you questions about the relationships you indicated—so be prepared with good answers. Some faculty may prefer that you write out why these linkages are important. The sloppy copy should now look like Figure 3.13.

Your explanations of the primary relationships between nursing diagnoses will be based on your knowledge of the disease process, as in the following examples.

Imbalanced Nutrition and ***Impaired Urinary Elimination:*** These two concepts are always linked in any disease. What goes in and is metabolized must come out in equal amounts or there will be a health problem. Metabolism is altered with diabetes because a lack of insulin causes blood glucose to rise, and excess glucose spills into the urine. As glucose is excreted, water is pulled out of the body by osmosis, creating an osmotic diuresis. Osmosis is the process by which a solution of higher concentration pulls water across a semi permeable membrane to equalize the concentrations on both sides of the membrane. Currently, the patient is making up

● Figure 3.13   Sloppy copy with links between nursing diagnoses.

for the losses that created a state of dehydration by retaining fluids. Thus, at this point, intake exceeds output.

Imbalanced Nutrition and ***Impaired Physical Mobility:*** Without adequate nutrition, the body becomes weak and debilitated, leading to impaired physical mobility.

Imbalanced Nutrition and ***Ineffective Peripheral Tissue Perfusion:*** High blood glucose levels damage peripheral blood vessels, which in turn leads to problems with tissue oxygenation and nerve damage, leading to hypertension, cardiovascular disease, peripheral neuropathies, nephropathies, foot ulcers, and infections.

Ineffective Peripheral Tissue Perfusion and ***Impaired Physical Mobility:*** Tissue perfusion

problems, treatment with an antihypertensive, and neuropathies all influence this patient's mobility, giving him an increased risk of falling and an increased risk of skin breakdown.

Deficient Knowledge, Anxiety, Ineffective Peripheral Tissue Perfusion, and ***Imbalanced Nutrition:*** Anxiety is common in newly diagnosed patients, no matter which health problem is involved. Anxiety may result from self-doubts about performing self-care and making lifestyle changes. Knowledge of the disease and treatments may serve to decrease patient anxiety. The patient will need to learn about the disease itself, including signs and symptoms, dietary management, blood glucose monitoring, insulin administration, exercise, and skin and foot care.

CHAPTER 3 SUMMARY

Important note: The diagnoses the night before clinical are primarily physiological, but should always include anticipated knowledge deficits and psychosocial and emotional problems, such as anxiety, if you have the assessment data to support them. The focus of the initial plan is based only on recorded data and perhaps a brief introduction to your patient and a brief talk with the staff nurse.

Typically, little is formally written about the psychosocial and cultural assessment unless you are in a psychiatric setting. The psychosocial and cultural assessment is much less formal than the physiological assessment in most care settings, including home care settings. You must spend time with the patient to do this assessment; then you can add psychosocial and cultural diagnoses to the concept care map on the day you care for the patient. This is the focus of Chapter 6.

The purpose of this chapter was to take you slowly through the first three steps of the concept map care planning process. After you gather clinical data, step 1 is to map the framework of propositions by noting the major medical diagnosis and the problems that result from that medical diagnosis. In step 2, organize the data into a hierarchy of subordinate concepts. This involves organizing abnormal physical assessment data, treatments, medications, diagnostic and laboratory tests, past medical problems and chronic illnesses, and emotional state as evidence to support the identification of problems from step 1. An important aspect of step 2 is the identification of key areas of assessment related to the primary medical diagnosis. Step 2 culminates in the final selection of nursing diagnoses based on the analysis of all available data. Step 3 involves the identification of meaningful associations between concepts on the map. The relationships between the nursing diagnoses are indicated with lines. The relationships you indicate must be accurate, meaningful, and complete; you should be prepared to explain why you believe a relationship exists between two connected diagnoses. In the Learning Activities, you will find two additional case studies in Figures 3.14 and 3.15 that you can use to practice steps 1, 2, and 3 of the concept care mapping process. Additional case studies can also be found on DavisPlus.

LEARNING ACTIVITIES

1. Patient case studies appear in Figures 3.14 and 3.15. Develop concept care maps for the data presented in these figures.

2. Compare concept care maps with your classmates.

3. During class, explain to your classmates why you believe relationships exist between nursing diagnoses you have connected with lines in step 3.

4. As homework, write out why you believe relationships exist between nursing diagnoses you have connected with lines in step 3, as was illustrated in the chapter under the subtitle of step 3: Mapping Cross-Links.

Student Name: **MAB**

1) Date of Care: **12/24**	2) Patient Initials: **AL**	3) Age: **78** (face sheet)	3) Growth and Development **Ego integrity vs. Despair**	4) Gender: **F** (face sheet)	5) Admission Date: (face sheet) **12/3**

6) Reason for hospitalization (face sheet): Describe reason for hospitalization: (expand on back of page) *Medical Dx:* **Breast Cancer** *Pathophysiology:* *All signs and symptoms: Highlight those your patient exhibits*	7) Chronic illnesses (physician's history and physical notes in chart; nursing intake assessment and Kardex) **NIDDM** **Hypertension** **MI 1994**
8) Surgical procedures (consent forms and Kardex): Describe surgical procedure (expand on back of page) Name of surgical procedure: **Mastectomy** *Describe surgery:* **Right modified radical mastectomy**	

9) ADVANCE DIRECTIVES (NURSE'S ADMISSION ASSESSMENTS):

Living will: ☐ Yes ☐ No	Power of attorney: ☐ Yes ☐ No	Do not resuscitate (DNR) order (Kardex): ☐ Yes ☐ No

10) LABORATORY DATA:

Test	Normal Values	Admission 12/3	Date/Time 12/4	Date/Time	Reason for Abnormal Values
White blood cells (WBCs)		5.6	4.8		
Red blood cells (RBCs)					
Hemoglobin (Hgb)		11.2	11		
Hematocrit (Hct)		33.2	33.1		
Platelets		259,000			
Prothrombin time (PT)					
International normalized ratio (INR)					
Activated partial thromboplastin time (Aptt)					
Sodium Na					
Potassium K		2.8	2.8		
Chloride Cl					
Glucose (FBS/BS)		230	235		
Hemoglobin A1C					
Cholesterol					
Blood Urea Nitrogen (BUN)					
Creatinine					
Urine analysis (UA)					
Pre-albumin					
Albumin					
Calcium Ca					
Phosphate					
Bilirubin					
Alkaline phosphatase					
SGOT-Serum glutamic-oxyloacetic transaminase					
AST-Serum glutamic pyruvic transaminase					
CK					
CK MB					
Troponin					
B-natriuretic peptide BNP					
pH					
pCO_2					
pO_2					
HCO_3					

11) DIAGNOSTIC TESTS

Chest x-ray:	EKG:	Other abnormal reports:
Sputum or Blood Culture:	Other:	Other:

● Figure 3.14 Patient profile database. Case Study 2: A surgical patient with a mastectomy.

12) MEDICATIONS

List medications and times of administration (medication administration record and check the drawer in the carts for spelling). Include over-the-counter (OTC) products/herbal medicines

Times Due	1000	0800	1000	1000
Brand Name		Lasix	Tenormin	Zoloft
Generic Name	heparin	furosemide	atenolol	sertraline
Dose	5000U	40mg	25mg	25mg
Administration Route	sq	po	po	po
Classification				
Action				
Reason This Patient is Receiving				
Pharmacokinetics	O P D 1/2 M E	O P D 1/2 M E	O P D 1/2 M E	O P D 1/2 M E
Contraindications				
Major Adverse Side Effects				
Nursing Implications				
Pt/Family Teaching				

Developed by P. Testa, YSU

Times Due	1000	1000	1000	q4h pm
Brand Name	Lanoxin	Ecotrin	K-dur	Tylenol
Generic Name	digoxin	aspirin	KCL	acetaminophen
Dose	01.25mg	1 tablet	20mg	650mg
Administration Route	po	po	po	po
Classification				
Action				
Reason This Patient is Receiving				
Pharmacokinetics	O P D 1/2 M E	O P D 1/2 M E	O P D 1/2 M E	O P D 1/2 M E
Contraindications				
Major Adverse Side Effects				
Nursing Implications				
Pt/Family Teaching				

Developed by P. Testa, YSU

ALLERGIES/PAINS

13) Allergies: **NKA** Type of Reaction: (medication administration record):	14) When was the last time pain medication given? (medication administration record) **Tylenol 6am (getting it sporadically)**
14) Where is the pain? **surgical incision** (nurse's notes)	14) How much pain is the patient in on a scale from 0-10? (nurse's notes, flow sheet): **5, confusion makes it unreliable**

TREATMENTS

15) List Treatments (Kardex): Rationale for treatments:
Dressing changes—sterile gauze & surgical bra, change qam
Ice to incision
Ted hose
IS q2h while awake
C&DB q2h while awake
I and O, & record q1h x 2

● Figure 3.14 Continued

16) Support services (Kardex) What do support services provide for the patient?

17) What does the consultant do for the patient?:

18) DIET/FLUIDS

Type of Diet (Kardex): **1800 ADA**	Restrictions (Kardex):	Gag reflex intact: ☐Yes ☐No	Appetite:☐Good ☐Fair ☒Poor	Breakfast **Eating Jello and tea only**	Lunch ____ %	Dinner ____ %

What type of diet is this?:

What types of foods are included in this diet and what foods should be avoided?:

Circle Those Problems That Apply:	
Prior 24 hours Fluid intake: (Oral & IV) **2100** Fluid output **1700** (flow sheet)	• Problems: swallowing, chewing, dentures (nurse's notes) • Needs assistance with feeding (nurse's notes) • Nausea or vomiting (nurse's notes) • Overhydrated or dehydrated (evaluate total intake and output on flow sheet
Tube feedings: Type and rate (Kardex)	• Belching: • Other:_____ **Dentures and needs assistance eating**

19) INTRAVENOUS FLUIDS (IV therapy record)

Type and Rate: **LR with 20 KCl 100/h**	IV dressing dry, no edema, redness of site: ☒ Yes ☐No	Other:

20) ELIMINATION (flow sheet)

Last bowel movement: **None since surgery**	Foley/condom catheter: ☐Yes ☒No

Circle Those Problems That Apply:

• Bowel: constipation, diarrhea, flatus, incontinence, belching
• Urinary: hesitancy, frequency, burning, incontinence, odor
• Other: _____
• What is causing the problem in elimination? _____

21) ACTIVITY (Kardex, flow sheet)

Ability to walk (gait):	Type of activity orders: **up as tolerated**	Use of assistance devices: cane, walker, crutches, prosthesis:	Falls-risk assessment rating: **7 high**
No. of side rails required (flow sheet) **4**	Restraints (flow sheet): ☒ Yes ☐No **vest, wrist**	Weakness ☒Yes ☐No	Trouble sleeping (nurse's notes): ☒Yes ☐No

What does activity order mean?: _____
Why isn't the patient up ad lib?: _____
Would the problem cause weakness?: _____

PHYSICAL ASSESSMENT DATA

22) BP (flow sheet): **137/72** **152/100**	2) TPR (flow sheet): **97-52-20** **97.8-80-20**	23) Height: __5'5"__ Weight: __190#__ (nursing intake assessments)

24) NEUROLOGICAL/MENTAL STATUS:

LOC: alert and oriented to person, place, time (A&O x 3), confused, etc. **Alert & oriented to person only, became confused evening after surgery**	Speech: clear, appropriate/inappropriate **inappropriate**
Pupils: PERRLA	Sensory deficits for vision/hearing/taste/ smell **glasses**

● Figure 3.14 Continued

25) MUSCULOSKELETAL STATUS:

Bones, joints, muscles (fractures, contractures, arthritis, spinal curvatures, etc):	Extremity (temperature, edema (pitting vs. nonpitting) & sensation)
Motor: ROM x 4 extremities	
Ted hose/plexi pulses/compression devices: type:	Casts, splint, collar, brace:

26) CARDIOVASCULAR SYSTEM:

Pulses (radial, pedal) (to touch or with Doppler):	Capillary refill (<3s): ☐ Yes ☐ No	
Neck vein (distention):	Sounds: S1, S2, regular, irregular: Apical rate: **80**	Any chest pain:

27) RESPIRATORY SYSTEM:

Depth, rate, rhythm: **20**	Use of accessory muscles:	Cyanosis:	Sputum color, amount:	Cough: productive nonproductive	Breath sounds: clear, rales, wheezes **Clear, decreased in bases**
Use of oxygen: nasal cannula, mask, trach collar:	Flow rate of oxygen:	Oxygen humidification: ☐ Yes ☐ No		Pulse oximeter: _____ % oxygen saturation	Smoking: ☐ Yes ☐ No

28) GASTROINTESTINAL SYSTEM

Abdominal pain, tenderness, guarding; distention, soft, firm: **Soft & nondistended**	Bowel sounds x 4 quadrants: **Active 4 quads**	NG tube: describe drainage
Ostomy: describe stoma site and stools:	Other:	

29) SKIN AND WOUNDS:

Color, turgor: **Pink, poor turgor**	Rash, bruises: **Dry and chapped**	Describe wounds (size, locations): **Red & edematous**	Edges approximated: ☒ Yes ☐ No	Type of wound drains: **JP #1 25 ml** **JP #2 100 ml**
Characteristics of drainage: **serosanguineous**	Dressings (clean, dry, intact): **Clean, dry, intact**	Sutures, staples, steri-strips, other:	Risk for pressure ulcer assessment rating:	Other:

30) EYES, EARS, NOSE, THROAT (EENT):

Eyes: redness, drainage, edema, ptosis	Ears: drainage	Nose: redness, drainage, edema	Throat: sore
Psychosocial and Cultural Assessment			
31) Religious preference (face sheet) **Catholic**	32) Marital status (face sheet) **Widowed**	33) Health care benefits and insurance (face sheet): **Medicare**	
34) Occupation (face sheet) **Housewife**	35) Emotional state (nurse's notes) **Anxious, wants to go home, very talkative, does not respond to questions appropriately**		

● Figure 3.14   Continued

Student Name: **BCD**

1) Date of Care: **2/5**	2) Patient Initials: **PUD**	3) Age: **55** (face sheet)	3) Growth and Development **Generativity vs. Stagnation**	4) Gender: **M** (face sheet)	5) Admission Date: (face sheet) **2/4**

6) Reason for hospitalization (face sheet): Describe reason for hospitalization: (expand on back of page) *Medical Dx:* **Arthritis, Chronic Pain right knee** *Pathophysiology:* *All signs and symptoms: Highlight those your patient exhibits*	7) Chronic illnesses (physician's history and physical notes in chart; nursing intake assessment and Kardex) **Hypertension**
8) Surgical procedures (consent forms and Kardex): Describe Surgical procedure (expand on back of page) Name of surgical procedure: **Right Knee Total Arthroplasty** *Describe surgery:*	

9) ADVANCE DIRECTIVES (NURSE'S ADMISSION ASSESSMENTS):

Living will: ☐ Yes ☐ No	Power of attorney: ☐ Yes ☐ No	Do not resuscitate (DNR) order (Kardex): ☐ Yes ☐ No

10) LABORATORY DATA:

Test	Normal Values	Admission 2/4	Date/Time	Date/Time	Reason for Abnormal Values
White blood cells (WBCs)		4.8			
Red blood cells (RBCs)					
Hemoglobin (Hgb)		12.5			
Hematocrit (Hct)		35.3			
Platelets		173,000			
Prothrombin time (PT)		11.5			
International normalized ratio (INR)					
Activated partial thromboplastin time (Aptt)		26.1			
Sodium Na					
Potassium K					
Chloride Cl					
Glucose (FBS/BS)					
Hemoglobin A1C					
Cholesterol					
Blood Urea Nitrogen (BUN)					
Creatinine					
Urine analysis (UA)					
Pre-albumin					
Albumin					
Calcium Ca					
Phosphate					
Bilirubin					
Alkaline phosphatase					
SGOT-Serum glutamic-oxyloacetic transaminase					
AST-Serum glutamic pyruvic transaminase					
CK					
CK MB					
Troponin					
B-natriuretic peptide BNP					
pH					
pCO_2					
pO_2					
HCO_3					

11) DIAGNOSTIC TESTS

Chest x-ray:	EKG:	Other abnormal reports:
Sputum or Blood Culture:	Other:	Other:

● Figure 3.15   Patient profile database. Case Study 3: A surgical patient with a knee replacement.

12) MEDICATIONS
List medications and times of administration (medication administration record and check the drawer in the carts for spelling). Include over-the-counter (OTC) products/herbal medicines.

Times Due	bid	qd	qd	q8h
Brand Name	K-dur	Hytrin	Colace	Kefzol
Generic Name	KCl	terazosin	docusate	cefazolin
Dose	20meq	5mg	100mg	1 g
Administration Route	po	po	po	po
Classification				
Action				
Reason This Patient is Receiving				
Pharmacokinetics	O P D 1/2 M E	O P D 1/2 M E	O P D 1/2 M E	O P D 1/2 M E
Contraindications				
Major Adverse Side Effects				
Nursing Implications				
Pt/Family Teaching				

Developed by P. Testa, YSU

Times Due	qd	q3-4h prn pain	q3-4h prn pain	q6h prn N?V
Brand Name	Lovenox	Demoral	Vicodin	Tigan
Generic Name	enoxaparin	meperidene	acetaminophen hydrocodone	trimethoben-zamid
Dose	30mg	75mg	500mg/5mg 1-2 tablets	200mg
Administration Route	sq	IM	po	IM
Classification				
Action				
Reason This Patient is Receiving				
Pharmacokinetics				
	O P D 1/2 M E	O P D 1/2 M E	O P D 1/2 M E	O P D 1/2 M E
Contraindications				
Major Adverse Side Effects				
Nursing Implications				
Pt/Family Teaching				

Developed by P. Testa, YSU

ALLERGIES/PAINS

13) Allergies: **sulfa, tetanus** Type of Reaction: (medication administration record):	14) When was the last time pain medication given? (medication administration record) **Darvocet 6am (getting it sporadically)**
14) Where is the pain? **incision** (nurse's notes)	14) How much pain is the patient in on a scale from 0-10? (nurse's notes, flow sheet): **8, decreased to 2 after meds**

TREATMENTS

15) List Treatments (Kardex): Rationale for treatments:

Dressing changes—begin po day 1 **Mini-pillow under ankle**
Ice to knee **Plexi pulses**
Foley **Overhead frame & trapeze**
IS q1h while awake with C&DB q2h while awake
CPM q shift for 3h

● Figure 3.15 Continued

16) Support services (Kardex) What do support services provide for the patient? **Physical Therapy to teach pt to use walker and CPM**
17) What does the consultant do for the patient?:

18) DIET/FLUIDS

Type of Diet (Kardex): **Regular**	Restrictions (Kardex):	Gag reflex intact: ☐Yes ☐No	Appetite:☐Good ☐Fair ☐Poor	Breakfast __75__ %	Lunch __50__ %	Dinner __75__ %
What type of diet is this?:						
What types of foods are included in this diet and what foods should be avoided?:						

Circle Those Problems That Apply:	
Prior 24 hours Fluid intake: (Oral & IV) **1040** Fluid output **975** (flow sheet)	• Problems: swallowing, chewing, dentures (nurse's notes) • Needs assistance with feeding (nurse's notes) • Nausea or vomiting (nurse's notes) • Overhydrated or dehydrated (evaluate total intake and output on flow sheet
Tube feedings: Type and rate (Kardex)	• Belching: • Other:_____

19) INTRAVENOUS FLUIDS (IV therapy record)

Type and Rate: **Autotransfusion, D5W 1/2 NS 1000 ml q 12h**	IV dressing dry, no edema, redness of site: ☒Yes ☐No	Other:

20) ELIMINATION (flow sheet)

Last bowel movement: **2/3**	Foley/condom catheter: ☒Yes ☐No **clear yellow urine**

Circle Those Problems That Apply:

• Bowel: constipation, diarrhea, flatus, incontinence, belching
• Urinary: hesitancy, frequency, burning, incontinence, odor
• Other: _____
• What is causing the problem in elimination? _____

21) ACTIVITY (Kardex, flow sheet)

Ability to walk (gait): **Unsteady**	Type of activity orders: **WBAT**	Use of assistance devices: cane, walker, crutches, prosthesis: **Walker**	Falls-risk assessment rating: **5 high**
No. of side rails required (flow sheet) **2**	Restraints (flow sheet): ☐Yes ☒No	Weakness ☒Yes ☐No	Trouble sleeping (nurse's notes): ☐Yes ☒No

What does activity order mean?: _____
Why isn't the patient up ad lib?: _____
Would the problem cause weakness?: _____

PHYSICAL ASSESSMENT DATA

22) BP (flow sheet): **124/66**	2) TPR (flow sheet): **36.6**	23) Height: __5'11"__ Weight: __202#__ (nursing intake assessments)

24) NEUROLOGICAL/MENTAL STATUS:

LOC: alert and oriented to person, place, time (A&O x 3) confused, etc. **A&O x 3**	Speech: clear, appropriate/inappropriate **clear**
Pupils: **PERRLA**	Sensory deficits for vision/hearing/taste/ smell **glasses**

● Figure 3.15 Continued

25) MUSCULOSKELETAL STATUS:

Bones, joints, muscles (fractures, contractures, arthritis, spinal curvatures, etc):	Extremity (temperature, edema (pitting vs. nonpitting) & sensation) **slight edema rt. Knee & lower leg**	
Motor: ROM x 4 extremities **decreased rt. knee**		
Ted hose/plexi pulses/compression devices: type: **Plexi pulses on at all times while in bed**	Casts, splint, collar, brace:	

26) CARDIOVASCULAR SYSTEM:

Pulses (radial, pedal) (to touch or with Doppler): **Pedals 3+ bilaterally**	Capillary refill (<3s): ☐ Yes ☐ No	
Neck vein (distention):	Sounds: S1, S2, regular, irregular: Apical rate:	Any chest pain:

27) RESPIRATORY SYSTEM:

Depth, rate, rhythm: **20**	Use of accessory muscles:	Cyanosis:	Sputum color, amount:	Cough: productive nonproductive	Breath sounds: clear, rales, wheezes **clear**
Use of oxygen: nasal cannula, mask, trach collar:	Flow rate of oxygen:	Oxygen humidification: ☐ Yes ☐ No		Pulse oximeter: _____ % oxygen saturation	Smoking: ☒ Yes ☐ No **history**

28) GASTROINTESTINAL SYSTEM

Abdominal pain, tenderness, guarding; distention, soft, firm: **Soft**	Bowel sounds x 4 quadrants: **+4 quads**	NG tube: describe drainage
Ostomy: describe stoma site and stools:	Other:	

29) SKIN AND WOUNDS:

Color, turgor:	Rash, bruises:	Describe wounds (size, locations): **Surgical incision bruised & edematous**	Edges approximated: ☒ Yes ☐ No	Type of wound drains: **Hemovac**
Characteristics of drainage: **Red 50cc**	Dressings (clean, dry, intact): **Clean, dry, intact**	Sutures, staples, steri-strips, other: **Sutures intact**	Risk for pressure ulcer assessment rating: **20 low risk**	Other:

30) EYES, EARS, NOSE, THROAT (EENT):

Eyes: redness, drainage, edema, ptosis	Ears: drainage	Nose: redness, drainage, edema	Throat: sore
Psychosocial and Cultural Assessment			
31) Religious preference (face sheet) **Presbyterian**	32) Marital status (face sheet) **Married**	33) Health care benefits and insurance (face sheet): **Aetna**	
34) Occupation (face sheet) **salesman**	35) Emotional state (nurse's notes) **calm, happy surgery is over**		

● Figure 3.15   Continued

REFERENCES

1. *Nursing-Scope and Standards of Practice*. 2nd ed. Silver Spring, Md: American Nurses Association; 2010.
2. Novak J, Gowin DB. *Learning How to Learn*. New York, NY: Cambridge University Press; 1984 (reprinted 2002).
3. Ausubel DP, Novak JD, Hanesian H. *Educational Psychology: A Cognitive View*. 2nd ed. New York, NY: Werbel and Peck; 1986. (classic reference)
4. Vallerand AH, Sanoski CA. *Davis's Drug Guide for Nurses*. 14th ed. Philadelphia, Pa: F.A. Davis; 2014.
5. Doenges ME, Moorhouse MF, Murr AC. *Nurse's Pocket Guide: Diagnoses, Interventions, and Rationales*. 13th ed. Philadelphia, Pa: F.A. Davis; 2013.
6. Brians LK, et al. The development of the RISK tool for fall prevention. *Rehabilitation Nursing*. 1991;16(2):67.
7. Braden B, Bergstrom N. In: Bryant RA, ed. *Acute and Chronic Wounds: Nursing Management*. St. Louis, Mo: Mosby; 1992.
8. NANDA International. *NANDA Nursing Diagnoses: Definitions and Classification,* 10th ed. *2015–2017*. Herdman TH, ed. Chichester, United Kingdom: Wiley-Blackwell; 2014.
9. Carpenito-Moyet LJ. *Handbook of Nursing Diagnosis*. 14th ed. Philadelphia, Pa: Lippincott; 2012.
10. Ackley BJ, Ladwig GB. *Nursing Diagnosis Handbook: An Evidence-Based Guide to Planning Care*. 10th ed. St. Louis, Mo: Elsevier/Mosby; 2013.
11. Venes D, et al, eds. *Taber's Cyclopedic Medical Dictionary*. 22nd ed. Philadelphia, Pa: F.A. Davis; 2013.
12. Ralph SS, Taylor CM. *Sparks and Taylor's Nursing Diagnosis Reference Manual*. 9th ed. Philadelphia, Pa: Lippincott; 2013.
13. Gordon M. *Manual of Nursing Diagnosis*. 13th ed. Sudbury, Mass: Jones and Bartlett; 2014.

NURSING STRATEGIES TO ATTAIN OUTCOMES: SO MANY PROBLEMS, SO LITTLE TIME

1. Identify the American Nurses Association (ANA) standards of professional nursing practice related to identifying patient outcomes and developing a plan that prescribes nursing strategies to attain expected outcomes.

2. Plan realistic and individualized goals, outcomes, and nursing strategies for each nursing diagnosis.

3. Include individualized physical and psychosocial nursing strategies in each plan of care.

4. Develop an individualized teaching plan for the day of care.

5. Describe the use of information from standardized care plans to select nursing strategies that are relevant to the assigned patient and situation.

6. Identify nursing strategies used to provide emotional support to patients and family members.

The focus of this chapter is step 4 of concept care mapping, which involves identifying therapeutic goals, outcomes, and nursing strategies needed to develop the plan of care. The American Nurses Association (ANA)[1] standards of professional nursing practice involving outcome identification and planning are standards 3 and 4. ANA standard 3 requires the nurse to identify expected outcomes that must be individualized for the patient and situation. For each nursing diagnosis, you must carefully identify the overall goal and specific patient outcomes. To do that, you need to know the progress that patients typically make in similar situations, and you need to know enough about the specifics of your patient's situation so that you can accurately predict outcomes. Ask yourself, "What will this patient do on the day I'm assigned to care for her to demonstrate that she is making progress and moving toward a healthier state?" Often, patients have multiple problems, and the outcome predictions may become difficult to make. Students commonly grow frustrated because a patient's condition changes between the time they gather the patient data and identify expected outcomes and the time they arrive on the unit to implement the plan of care. In the meantime, the patient's condition may have changed for better or worse, and the outcomes you anticipated and wrote on your plan of care may need to be revised. Sometimes the patient may have been transferred or even discharged.

ANA standard 4 requires the nurse to develop a plan of care that prescribes nursing strategies to attain the expected outcomes. You must plan for the patient's physical and emotional care, and you must know what each nursing strategy is intended to accomplish regarding the expected outcomes for the patient. In addition, your plan of care must include the development of a specific teaching plan. The purpose of this chapter is to help develop your critical thinking process in prioritizing problems, developing patient goals and outcomes, and selecting nursing strategies to attain those goals and outcomes. You will also work on developing a teaching plan for the diabetic patient introduced in earlier chapters.

Step 4: Thinking Critically About Patient Outcomes and Nursing Strategies

Review the concept care map shown in Figure 4.1. It is the one developed in Chapter 3, with a few details added. This concept care map is prioritized and ready for use in the clinical setting. Note the patient's problem areas: nutrition, urinary elimination, mobility, anxiety, tissue perfusion, and knowledge deficits. It is important to be able to arrange problem areas in priority order, to guide your nursing strategies as you deliver care to your patients and their families.

Identifying Priority Problem No. 1

Find the box on the concept care map that has the most supporting data in it and label it "Problem No. 1." Usually, the most important diagnosis has the most supporting data and is the priority for planning care. In this example, *Imbalanced Nutrition: Less Than Body Requirements* is the priority diagnosis. Given the pathophysiology of diabetes mellitus, it makes sense that the patient's nutritional state is going to be highly disrupted; the goal will be to improve the patient's nutritional status. To attain this goal, you need to determine expected outcomes on the day you are assigned to care for the patient, think critically to determine nursing strategies, and document the problems, goal, outcomes, and strategies.

Assigning Outcomes

As a general goal, the patient would be expected to continue improving his nutritional status. It is important to assess his progress toward this goal and to discern what needs to be accomplished for him to achieve a healthier state.

For this particular patient, the last known blood glucose level was 110 mg/dL. Normal blood glucose levels are 70 to 110 mg/dL; therefore, a major predicted outcome is that the patient will maintain his blood sugar between 80 mg/dL and 110 mg/dL by eating his 1800-calorie diet and taking insulin injections as scheduled.

Nursing Strategies

What must you do to make sure the patient attains this outcome? Use the patient data in the box you labeled with the diagnosis of *Imbalanced Nutrition: Less Than Body Requirements.* The data on your concept care map give many clues as to what your strategies will involve:

- Assess the abdomen.
- Assess the patient for hyperglycemia and obtain a medication order to give additional insulin if indicated.
- Assess the patient's blood glucose with the glucometer.
- Monitor the patient's appetite and encourage him to eat his meals.
- Administer his insulin injections as scheduled.
- Watch for signs and symptoms of hypoglycemia, especially if the patient's intake is not sufficient.

#6
Key Problem
Impaired Urinary Elimination

Intake = 2200
Output = 1800
Polyuria
3+sugar

I don't know how this fits with the problems.

Acetaminophen?
Widower?

#1
Key Problem
Imbalanced Nutrition: Less than Body Requirements

Polydipsia
Intake = 2200
Output = 1800
Weakness
174#
Humulin N
Glucose (450)120
Glyco Hgb = 12%
Cholesterol 240
Glucometer
1800 ADA no sugar added

#2
Key Problem
Acute Anxiety

Expresses concern over injections and diet
New Diagnosis

Reason For Needing Health Care:
Medical Diagnosis/Surgical Procedure:
Newly Diagnosed Diabetes

Key Assessments:
Signs and symptoms of hypoglycemia & hyperglycemia, monitor blood glucose, food intake & VS

#4
Key Problem
Ineffective Peripheral Tissue Perfusion

138.92
Valsartan (Diovan)
VS qid
98.4-77-18
Potential Skin Breakdown

#3
Key Problem
Deficient Knowledge

Diagnosis
Medications
Diet
Skin Care
Foot Care
Exercise

#5
Key Problem
Impaired Physical Mobility

Risk for Falls-4
OOB/chair
Weakness

● Figure 4.1   Concept care map for a diabetic patient, with problems prioritized.

Continuous assessment is the first priority when you list nursing strategies used to attain outcomes. It is critically imperative to focus on the primary system of the body affected—in this case, the gastrointestinal (GI) system. Therefore, the first strategy that should be listed is always the assessment you intend to perform to monitor the physical signs and symptoms of the altered health state represented by the nursing diagnosis. With the diagnosis of *Imbalanced Nutrition: Less Than Body Requirements,* the basic GI assessment includes bowel sounds,

abdominal tenderness, distention, and bowel movements. Assessments include monitoring for hypoglycemia and hyperglycemia.

Take another look at the data in the box for nutrition. What about the polydipsia and 2200-cc intake and 1800-cc output? You will need to continue monitoring the patient's intake and output. Remember that polydipsia and polyuria are classic signs of hyperglycemia, and that this patient became dehydrated before he was hospitalized. Currently, his intake exceeds his output because his body is trying to make up for the fluid loss.

The patient's weakness stems from lack of food and from dehydration. Therefore, you will need to monitor his appetite and encourage him to consume his 1800-calorie diet, no sugar added. Calories and food types will need to be regulated carefully against the amount of insulin administered and the patient's level of exercise. Usually it takes several days of blood glucose monitoring and insulin adjustment before a patient's daily diet, exercise, and insulin patterns can be stabilized. In regulating a diabetic patient's condition, it is imperative that there be a counterbalance among calories consumed, insulin dosages, and exercise.

Keep in mind that this patient's weakness is a safety risk for falls. Caution is warranted when transferring him and helping him ambulate. As he continues to progress, he should become stronger. Assess his weakness level when you first meet him on the day of care by asking him how much help he needs walking. His risk for falls may also be partly related to his antihypertensive therapy and his age. Antihypertensive drugs commonly cause orthostatic hypotension, which is a drop in blood pressure that causes symptoms of lightheadedness when the patient changes positions, particularly when moved from lying down to sitting or standing up. As people age, the valves inside leg veins commonly weaken, which can lead to pooling of blood in the periphery and may further contribute to orthostatic hypotension. To determine the possible effects of orthostatic hypotension on your patient, check his blood pressure and pulse while he sits on the side of his bed. Also, before you help him up, ask him whether he gets dizzy when he stands up. That way, you will reduce the patient's risk of falls and possibly becoming injured.

The rest of the data in the *Imbalanced Nutrition: Less Than Body Requirements* box on your concept care map address additional blood work to check glycohemoglobin (Hgb A1c) and cholesterol. These blood samples would not be drawn every day. You must plan to check the results of any blood work that is ordered and promptly report abnormal values to your clinical faculty, the agency nurse, and the patient's doctor. For example, the doctor may have ordered that electrolytes be drawn. Review those reports as soon as they become available.

Always be aware of the time that any blood work is done and the time the reports should be available. Sometimes blood samples get lost. If the reports are not available as scheduled, you may need to contact the laboratory to make sure the blood sample was received and is being processed.

Writing Problems, Goals, Outcomes, and Strategies

A blank sample format to guide you in writing out problems, goals, outcomes, and nursing strategies is shown in Figure 4.2. Figure 4.3 contains goals, outcomes, and strategies for this diabetic patient scenario. You have identified nutrition as the top priority for your patient, so write it as Problem No. 1 and list the goals and expected outcomes under this problem. In the column labeled "Nursing Strategies," write brief notes of all the things you are planning to do, based on what you believe to be important from your analysis of the information in the nutrition box. The right-hand column on the form is reserved for direct observations made of the patient during the clinical day. You will record the patient's responses to each of the listed nursing strategies and thus use this column to evaluate the patient. This process is explained further in Chapter 5.

The nursing strategies listed so far can be classified as physically supportive of the patient. Nurses perform physical assessments (gastrointestinal system), use equipment to monitor patients (glucometer), monitor laboratory and diagnostic tests (blood glucose), administer medications (insulin), and perform treatments (none for this particular diagnosis).

Identifying Priority Problem No. 2

Look back at the concept care map again. *Anxiety* and *Deficient Knowledge* are very important interacting diagnoses. Recall that there is a direct line drawn between Anxiety and Deficient Knowledge, indicating the relationship between these nursing diagnoses. The goals are to decrease anxiety and increase knowledge of diabetes. When anxiety is decreased, the patient will be able to learn better, and when he has knowledge of self-care, he will have less anxiety about his ability to perform

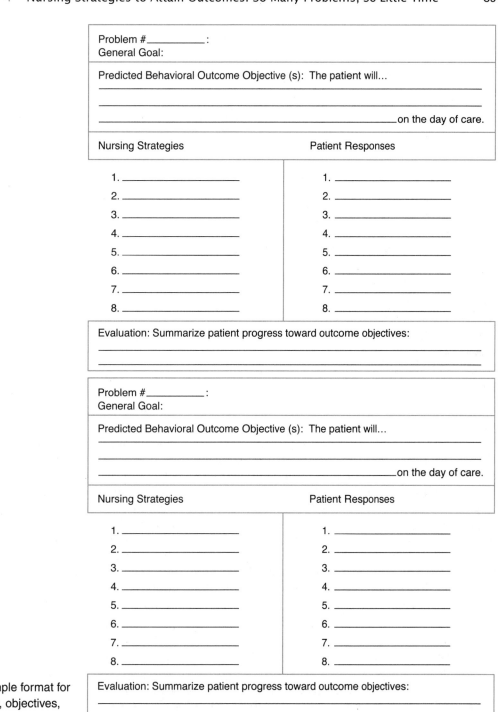

Problem #_____ :
General Goal:

Predicted Behavioral Outcome Objective (s): The patient will...
_____
_____
_____on the day of care.

Nursing Strategies	Patient Responses
1. _____	1. _____
2. _____	2. _____
3. _____	3. _____
4. _____	4. _____
5. _____	5. _____
6. _____	6. _____
7. _____	7. _____
8. _____	8. _____

Evaluation: Summarize patient progress toward outcome objectives:
_____
_____

Problem #_____ :
General Goal:

Predicted Behavioral Outcome Objective (s): The patient will...
_____
_____
_____on the day of care.

Nursing Strategies	Patient Responses
1. _____	1. _____
2. _____	2. _____
3. _____	3. _____
4. _____	4. _____
5. _____	5. _____
6. _____	6. _____
7. _____	7. _____
8. _____	8. _____

Evaluation: Summarize patient progress toward outcome objectives:
_____
_____

● Figure 4.2   Sample format for writing problems, goals, objectives, strategies, responses, and summary.

self-care. Anxiety is a common emotional reaction to the stress of illness. For this patient, anxiety may result from his recognition that he must make changes in his lifestyle and that he lacks the confidence and knowledge to make those changes. Consequently, his anxiety must be assessed and reduced before teaching will be successful.

Therefore, anxiety reduction takes priority over patient education. Label it Problem No. 2, as shown in Figure 4.4. Patients are not able to

---

Problem #__1__ : Imbalanced Nutrition: Less than body requirements
General Goal: To improve the patient's nutritional status

Predicted Behavioral Outcome Objective (s): The patient will…maintain his blood glucose between 80 and 120 mg/dl by eating his 1800-calorie ADA diet and administering insulin injections as scheduled… on the day of care.

Nursing Strategies	Patient Responses
1. Assess abdomen: bowel sounds, tenderness, distention, BMs	1.
2. Assess blood glucose with glucometer at 0800 and 1100	2.
3. Assess S/S of hypoglycemia and hyperglycemia	3.
4. Monitor appetite—1800 cal ADA, no sugar added	4.
5. Measure fluid intake and output	5.
6. Administer insulin on time	6.
7. Check for additional blood work	7.
8. Monitor patient for orthostatic hypotension and weakness	8.
9. Ambulate carefully to avoid falls	9.

● Figure 4.3   Problem No. 1.

concentrate and learn when their anxiety is high. The net result of too much anxiety is usually impaired cognitive function, which simply means that the brain does not work as well. Short-term memory, concentration, and abstract thought can be altered in high-anxiety states. Patients' thoughts are blocked; patients may appear confused and forgetful, and they may have difficulty concentrating. All of these factors contribute to a decreased learning ability. A little anxiety, however, can be motivational. If the patient is slightly anxious, his senses are on full alert, and he can use the increased alertness and energy to his advantage to learn about self-care. The goal is to decrease the patient's anxiety but not to completely obliterate it.

Once you believe the problem is anxiety, use a basic care planning book to confirm the diagnosis. Look up the nursing diagnosis *Anxiety* to determine its behavioral, affective, physiological, and cognitive defining characteristics. For example, a partial list from NANDA[2] of the defining characteristics of anxiety includes insomnia, fidgeting, poor eye contact, and restlessness. Some affective signs of anxiety are irritability, uncertainty, and feelings of inadequacy. Physiological

---

Problem #__2__ : Anxiety
General Goal: Decrease Anxiety

Predicted Behavioral Outcome Objective (s): The patient will…verbalize concerns about his disease and the changes that must be made in his lifestyle… on the day of care.

Nursing Strategies	Patient Responses
1. Assess current level of anxiety	1.
2. Use empathy	2.
3. Use therapeutic touch	3.
4. Use therapeutic humor	4.

● Figure 4.4   Problem No. 2.

signs include facial tension and increased heart rate and blood pressure. Among the cognitive signs are forgetfulness and impaired attention. The NANDA reference lists 74 defining characteristics for anxiety that should be assessed. If you assess each of the 74 characteristics of anxiety, you almost always find that a patient will be displaying some of these signs. In working with every patient, always assess anxiety. Anxiety results in painful emotions that always accompany physical and mental illness.

The anticipated outcome for an anxious patient is for him to verbalize concerns and express himself. Nurses need to plan specific strategies to provide emotional support to patients and family members. Appropriate nursing strategies for providing emotional support include the use of empathy, comfort touch, and therapeutic humor to facilitate ventilation of feelings and thus relieve anxiety.

Empathy is a very important strategy to learn for dealing with patients' painful emotional responses. The classic emotions of sadness, fear, and anger are prevalent during illness. Without release, emotional feelings of sadness can progress to clinical depression; specific fears can progress to diffuse anxiety; and anger may be manifested as hostility and resentment.

Allow the patient to have an emotional release by acknowledging and accepting his emotions and by encouraging him to express those emotions. Do not pretend that his emotions do not exist. Do not criticize emotions. Do not try to rationalize emotions. Do not try to change or fix emotions. At first, the person may yell or blame. He may placate and cry. Or he may be sarcastic and make jokes about his problems. After this period of ventilation, however, he may be able to express his frustrations with his current situation and begin to problem-solve.

The strategy of *touch* can be used to decrease the patient's response to anxiety. Carefully monitor the patient's responses to touch. Touch needs to be related to the context of the situation. Caring touch includes holding the patient's hand, placing an arm around his shoulders, and giving him a hug or a pat on the back. Touch can be used to support, reassure, and raise spirits. *Protective touch* is used when patient safety is a primary concern. A confused patient may be restrained and sedated to make sure he will not pull on vital tubes or fall out of bed. When

applying restraints, use caring touch at the same time. *Task touch* involves physical assessment and procedural treatments that must be done. Be gentle and careful with task touches and overlap them with caring touches.

The strategy of *therapeutic humor* may be used by nurses to help reduce mild anxiety and put people at ease. When people can see the absurdity in a situation and laugh at it, they can distance themselves from threatening problems. Humor is an effective coping mechanism that helps to reframe reality and reduce negative feelings. It facilitates the experience of relief from painful emotions. It is important not to be insulting when using humor, and to assess the patient carefully for physical and emotional discomforts before using humor in professional relationships. Additional strategies are listed in Box 4.1. Learning how to gain the cooperation and respect of patients when you are a rookie nursing student is covered in detail in Schuster and Nykolyn's book *Communication for Nurses: How to Prevent Harmful Events and Promote Patient Safety.*[3]

Identify Priority Problem No. 3

The third-priority problem for this patient is **Deficient Knowledge** of self-care and management of diabetes. Label it Problem No. 3 on your concept care map. It is a nursing responsibility to educate each patient about self-care and to include significant others in the teaching. According to data you have collected for your concept care map, this patient is most concerned about injections and diet. One of your first educational strategies may be to assess his knowledge of injections, diet, and other self-care activities (Fig. 4.5). Also ask your patient's staff nurse what information she has attempted to teach him and how he has responded to teaching.

As you collected patient data, there was no mention in the patient's records that he had seen a diabetes educator or attended classes. Find out what resources are available to bridge the gap between what he knows and what he needs to learn. Check to see what types of classes are available to the patient, whether the dietitian has been to talk to him, and whether a diabetes educator is available.

Each patient (and significant other) needs a teaching plan centered on the day of care. This

Box 4.1   NURSING STRATEGIES TO PROVIDE EMOTIONAL SUPPORT

Expressions of Sadness and Grief

Tears and crying are very important therapeutic resources that can be used to facilitate healing and well-being. Tears are a natural way of releasing tension that comes from sadness, grief, anger, and fear. Nursing a patient with a loss involves allowing the patient to experience an emotional release through tears. Avoid expressing disapproval or minimizing the cause of crying, and do not offer false hope or make promises that you cannot keep to make the crying stop. Listen supportively and empathetically to the patient's and family's verbalizations of emotional pain.

Building Self-Esteem

Self-esteem is the value a person places on himself and affects the way he interacts with others. Health problems commonly lower self-esteem. Those with low self-esteem may have feelings of isolation, helplessness, incompetence, or being unloved. To build self-esteem, define clear and realistic goals, help patients to think clearly, give positive feedback, encourage positive self-affirmations, and use visualization exercises.

Anticipatory Guidance

Nurses use anticipatory guidance to guide patients through uncomfortable procedures. Talk to your patients and explain the sensations they will be feeling, so they know what to expect and their anxiety will be reduced. For example, when giving an IM injection, say something like, "First I'll palpate and find the right spot. Then you will feel me wiping you off. Then you will feel a pinch and a little burning. It's the medication. All done. I'm massaging the site a little."

Reminiscing and Life Review

When using reminiscing, the nurse encourages the patient to recall and talk about life experiences. Reminiscing can be helpful in resocializing people and building relationships, while the life review helps people to make sense of their lives and to see their lives as unique stories. Nurses implement reminiscence or life review to help patients deal with crises and losses, to prevent and reduce depression, and to increase life satisfaction.

Distraction

Distraction is a technique used to take a patient's mind off what is bothering her. The patient may be nervously waiting to have a procedure done. She is prepared for it as well as she can be, so you make small talk about whatever interests her. This distraction also works when you are trying to get a slightly confused patient to cooperate with you. For example, say you have a slightly confused elderly patient who is demanding to go for a walk right now, despite having an NG tube, catheters, and IV lines. Although you may need to use light restraints, you may also be able to distract the patient from her demand by getting her interested in the television, a magazine, or a conversation.

Problem-Solving and Decision Making

Nurses commonly help patients solve problems and make decisions. The steps of the problem-solving or decision-making process include identifying the problem, searching for information about the problem, identifying options, examining the pros and cons of each option, choosing an option, developing a plan of action, implementing the plan, and evaluating the effects.

Source: Schuster P. *Communication: The Key to the Therapeutic Relationship.* Philadelphia, Pa: F.A. Davis; 2000.

Problem #__3__: Deficient knowledge General Goal: Increase knowledge
Predicted Behavioral Outcome Objective (s): The patient will…decide in collaboration with the nurse what aspects of diabetic teaching protocol he would like to focus on during…the day of care.

Nursing Strategies	Patient Responses
1. Assess current level of knowledge and establish what the patient most wants to learn about during the day of care	1.
2. Assess resources availabe for teaching, such as diabetic educator, dietitian, programs, or movies	2.

3. See teaching plan for:
  –what diabetes is and how it affects
    health (signs and symptoms)
  –Medications
  –Diet
  –Skin care
  –Exercise/activity
	3.

● Figure 4.5   Problem No. 3.

diabetic patient needs to know about his diagnosis, medications, diet, exercise, and skin care. He cannot possibly learn all of that in one day, but you must develop a general teaching plan before meeting with the patient.

To determine the content of your teaching plan, review a standardized nursing care plan book or computer program for educating patients about major diseases. While obtaining your patient assignment at the health-care agency, get any available teaching aids about his health problems. Read them carefully so you understand the basics of what the patient needs to know. From these resources, pick out the essential information that is pertinent to teach your patient.

Identify Priority Problem No. 4

Review your concept care map and look at the remaining diagnoses to select the problem of the fourth priority. The box with the diagnosis *Ineffective Peripheral Tissue Perfusion* contains more patient profile data than the boxes with *Impaired Physical Mobility* and *Impaired Urinary Elimination,* so you can label it Problem No. 4. The pathophysiology of diabetes affects the circulation; many diabetics have a history of hypertension. Specifically, diabetes speeds

up degeneration of the arteries and veins, and fat deposits build up in the blood vessels, leading to atherosclerosis and hypertension. Atherosclerosis is the cause of coronary artery disease (heart attacks), cerebrovascular disease (strokes), and peripheral vascular disease (arterial and venous ulcerations). Peripheral vascular disease has many implications for diabetics. With inadequate tissue perfusion, tissues will break down and pressure ulcers will form. Nerve degeneration also occurs in the periphery. This is termed *diabetic neuropathy* and results in pain, tingling, and burning in the legs. Neuropathy progresses to a lack of sensation in the legs as the disease worsens.

Therefore, the general goal is to maintain optimal tissue perfusion and circulation (Fig. 4.6). Specific outcomes include keeping the patient's vital signs close to normal and avoiding skin breakdown. The first strategy is always assessment. You will assess his vital signs, and will assess his circulation by checking capillary refill and peripheral pulses. You will also assess for skin breakdown and pressure ulcers. Other strategies include encouraging supervised ambulation, helping the patient into a chair, and encouraging the patient to perform range-of-motion exercises to improve circulation to his limbs and prevent skin breakdown.

Problem #__4__: Ineffective Peripheral Tissue Perfusion General Goal: Maintain optimal tissue perfusion and circulation	
Predicted Behavioral Outcome Objective (s): The patient will…have vital signs remaining close to normal, no skin breakdown, moves safely from bed to chair…on the day of care.	
Nursing Strategies	Patient Responses
1. Assess vital signs	1.
2. Assess peripheral pulses and capillary refill	2.
3. Assess skin for pressure sore	3.
4. Give valsartan, assess BP/P prior to administrations	4.
5. ROM extremities q2h if in bed	5.
6. Walk w/assistance	6.
7. Chair x 2	7.

● Figure 4.6   Problem No. 4.

Identifying Priority Problems No. 5 and No. 6

The two remaining diagnoses that have not been directly addressed are *Impaired Physical Mobility* and *Impaired Urinary Elimination.* These diagnoses are of equal importance and have been labeled Problem No. 5 and Problem No. 6 on the concept care map. It does not matter which is Problem 5 and which is Problem 6, as long as both are recognized as problems.

The goal with *Impaired Physical Mobility* is to prevent complications of immobility and to prevent falls. The patient outcomes are to sit in a chair with assistance, to perform range-of-motion exercises, and to ambulate as much as tolerated. Nursing strategies to attain these outcomes have been covered for Problems 1 and 4. Specifically, you will monitor the patient for orthostatic hypotension and weakness, and you will carefully assist the patient with ambulation, to avoid falls. You will also help the patient sit in a chair and perform range-of-motion exercises.

The goal for *Impaired Urinary Elimination* is to maintain normal urinary elimination. Outcomes include intake and output approaching normal values and the patient having no polyuria. Nursing strategies are covered under Problem 1 and include measuring fluid intake and output and monitoring for signs and symptoms of hyperglycemia and hypoglycemia.

The goals and outcomes for *Impaired Physical Mobility* and *Impaired Urinary Elimination* are shown in Figure 4.7. There is no need to copy nursing strategies that you have already specified into this summary. Instead, refer to the nursing strategies covered under previous nursing diagnoses.

Your basic care map is now complete, with goals, outcomes, and nursing strategies. You can carry the concept care map, complete with goals, outcomes, nursing strategies, and teaching plan in your pocket on the clinical units and use it during the implementation phase of the nursing process. Be prepared to discuss with your clinical faculty the rationales for each of the nursing strategies you identified. Although the basic care map is complete, you still need to develop a teaching plan. What follows is a discussion of one method for developing a teaching plan.

Developing a Mini–Teaching Plan Using METHOD

The last section of this chapter focuses on developing a one-page mini–individualized teaching plan with specific content and teaching methods. Box 4.2 shows an outline that you can use to develop a one-page mini–teaching plan. This outline focuses on key information that all patients and significant others need to know about the specific disease and its treatments.

Problem #__5__ : Impaired Physical Mobility General Goal: Prevent complications of immobility, prevent falls	
Predicted Behavioral Outcome Objective (s): The patient will...ambulate to chair and walk with steady gait, does range of motion exercises...on the day of care.	
Nursing Strategies	Patient Responses
1. Covered under Nutrition and Altered tissue perfusion	

Problem #__6__ : Impaired Urinary Elimination General Goal: Maintain normal urinary elimination	
Predicted Behavioral Outcome Objective (s): The patient will...have intake and output approaching normal values, no polyuria...on the day of care.	
Nursing Strategies	Patient Responses
1. Covered under Nutrition	

● Figure 4.7   Problems No. 5 and No. 6.

The key teaching areas are structured around the acronym METHOD.[3-5]

Using the acronym METHOD will help you remember key items to cover in every teaching plan you construct. Teaching is an essential component of all care planning. Students are required to come to clinical prepared to teach whatever is appropriate for the clinical day. If you are assigned to a preoperative patient, focus on preoperative teaching. If you are assigned to a first-day surgical patient, focus teaching on the first day after surgery. Focus on discharge teaching if the patient is being prepared to go home while you are taking care of him.

M is for Medications

Write the name (generic and brand name) and key action of each drug. Write one sentence for each drug that represents how you would explain it to your patient in words the patient and significant others can understand. Avoid using medical terminology from your drug guides. Use medical terminology only when explaining a drug's actions and side effects to your clinical faculty as you are preparing the drugs for administration. For example, write:

> ▸ "This is an antibiotic for your infection."
> ▸ "This is a blood thinner to prevent clots."

> ▸ "This is your pain pill."
> ▸ "This is your insulin to control your blood sugar."

Details about side effects are not necessary unless the patient is going home with the drug or is asking for more specific information. If he is going home with the drug, write the basics of what you will say in simple terms, with as few words as possible. For example, "Take Tylenol (acetaminophen) if you need something for discomfort. Don't take aspirin, because it is a blood thinner" or "Take your antibiotic three times a day: when you get up, in the afternoon, and at night before bed. Take the entire prescription. Don't stop before it's finished, even if you feel better. Take it with food if your stomach gets upset." Write down information if the patient is being discharged, so that he will have reminders when he is home of what is to be done and why.

E is for Environment

Environment includes the home or health-care agency environment, financial considerations, and social support. Review standardized nursing care plan guides and nursing texts to determine how the patient and significant others may need

Box 4.2   METHOD DAILY TEACHING PLAN

Patient Name

Diagnosis

Teaching Techniques

M (Medications):

E (Environment):

T (Treatments):

H (Health Knowledge of Disease):

O (Outpatient/Inpatient Referrals):

D (Diet):

to modify the home environment. Assess the patient's home situation, and intervene if needed. Determine whether the patient has the financial resources to implement the treatment plan, and intervene if necessary. Find out whether the patient has significant others to assist with care if needed. If significant others are not available, contacts with community agencies may be necessary to assist the patient in the adjustment to returning home. Also consider what you must do to provide a safe environment in the healthcare setting. For example, does the patient need the furniture rearranged so he may safely get up to a chair or walk to the bathroom? Is the call light in reach, is the bed down, are the side rails up, and are the wheels locked on the patient's bed? Patients and family members must be taught how to arrange their environments to prevent accidents.

T is for Treatments

Explain the purpose of each treatment and the correct techniques for performing treatments that will continue at home. For example, explain skin care procedures or wound care. Write down specifically what the patient needs to do. If written guidelines are available, highlight the most important things for the patient to remember. Exercise or activity guidelines may also be considered a treatment. Each patient must be aware of what activities are and are not permitted and how to develop and maintain an exercise routine. Many diabetic patients will be instructed to increase their walking gradually until they are walking for 30 minutes every day.

H is for Health Knowledge of Disease

Write down the effects of the patient's disease, signs and symptoms that he should watch for, and any changes that should prompt him to call the physician or nurse practitioner. For example, write down what the patient should watch for regarding signs and symptoms of an infection in a wound, a urine infection, or whatever is applicable to the patient's specific problems.

O is for Outpatient/Inpatient Referrals

Write a sentence to explain inpatient diagnostic tests or procedures using nonmedical terms. For outpatient referrals, list support groups, home health agencies, and dates and times of office appointments. Check with the staff nurse assigned to your patient during your assigned clinical day to find out the physician's usual routine for patients after discharge. Also, read the discharge orders.

D is for Diet

Write down the patient's appropriate diet and restrictions. Obtain examples of typical menus from the dietitian. Write down a list of foods that the patient can eat and foods that he should avoid, as applicable.

Sample METHOD Plan for a Diabetic Patient

For your diabetic patient, the METHOD teaching plan will result from a synthesis of concept care map data, standardized teaching plans, and education materials for diabetic patients. You will need to review a standardized teaching plan for diabetics, standardized patient information on insulin, standardized samples of the 1800-calorie American Diabetic Association (ADA) diet, and patient education booklets on diabetes. The following section walks you through the construction of a METHOD teaching plan for this patient.

Medications

Three drugs are listed on your concept care map: Humulin N, valsartan, and acetaminophen. Based on information you obtain from drug references, your patient teaching information about the patient's medications may look like what appears in Box 4.3. It is formatted using the actual words you might say to the patient. Keep in mind that although this section of the teaching plan is written in language that you plan to use as you teach the patient, the plan is actually for your use and not to be given to the patient. Naturally, you should be prepared to discuss the details of your teaching plan with your clinical faculty before giving a drug or even giving the patient this information. You should also be prepared to give the patient more information if he asks for it.

Environment

Your patient is an 80-year-old widower. He has insurance. To fill out this section of the teaching plan, assess him further to find out about his level of social support. Does he have family members or significant others to assist him at home and take him to follow-up appointments or diabetic education classes? Does he drive? While in the hospital, what special assistance did he need in his environment that he will still need at home? For example, does he need to be assisted with ambulation until his strength returns? He needs to be taught his activity restrictions while hospitalized. Therefore, the teaching plan could include the notations specified under Health Knowledge of Disease included in Box 4.3.

Box 4.3   SAMPLE METHOD DAILY TEACHING PLAN

Patient Name: ET
Diagnosis: Newly diagnosed Diabetes
Teaching Techniques: Give explanations, one-on-one discussion, demonstrations
M (Medications): Humulin N (NPH, human insulin) insulin: "This drug is to control blood glucose levels. Watch for signs and symptoms of hypoglycemia and hyperglycemia. Onset (1 to 2 hours), peak (6 to 12 hours), and duration (up to 24 hours). Take this drug each morning, 30 minutes before breakfast. If you do not eat as scheduled and in the amounts specified in your diet plan, you will probably have a hypoglycemic reaction in mid- to late afternoon (6 to 12 hours after you've taken the drug)."

Valsartan (Diovan): "This drug is to control your blood pressure. Watch for signs of low blood pressure. Get up slowly and sit on the side of the bed to avoid dizziness. Check your blood pressure and pulse."

Acetaminophen (Tylenol): "Take this drug in recommended amounts for aches and general discomfort; don't take aspirin, because aspirin causes blood thinning and could upset your stomach."

E (Environment): Assess patient for social supports to help him with self-care and transportation. Teach patient activity limitations while the patient is in the hospital, and find out activity prescription after discharge. Create an environment of trust and support so the patient can learn effectively.

T (Treatments): Demonstrate use of Accu-Chek or have patient do procedure if ready. Use patient teaching aid booklet and video if available.

Demonstrate insulin injection or have patient self-administer if ready. Demonstrate care of equipment. Use patient teaching aid booklet and video if available.

Describe skin care, wound care (if appropriate), and daily care of feet using teaching aids such as booklets or videos. Highlight information in patient teaching pamphlets: Use mild soap and lukewarm water. Use lotions to keep skin soft. Protect skin by using gloves while working and sunscreen while outdoors. Treat injuries immediately with soap, warm water, and dry sterile bandage. See physician or nurse practitioner if cuts do not heal or if they become infected (red, throbbing, warm, with swelling or pus).

Explain activity limitations and have patient reiterate. "You will be out of bed to sit in a chair and walk with assistance today. Until your strength returns, you will need assistance to prevent falls."

Box 4.3 SAMPLE METHOD DAILY TEACHING PLAN—cont'd

H (Health Knowledge of Disease): "Hypoglycemia may be caused by taking in too much insulin, missing or delaying meals, exercising or working more than usual, or getting an infection or illness. It can develop rapidly, in 15 minutes to 1 hour. Symptoms include sweating, dizziness, shaking, hunger, or restlessness; numbness or tingling of the lips, tongue, hands, or feet; slurred speech, headache, or blurred vision. Carry candy or fruit juice with you and eat or drink it if you feel a hypoglycemic reaction coming. When the reaction is over, eat a serving of a slowly digested food such as cottage cheese, drink milk, or have your scheduled meal or snack to prevent a second drop in blood sugar.

"Hyperglycemia can be caused by omitting insulin or taking less than prescribed, eating more than the prescribed diet, or experiencing a great deal of stress. Illnesses with fever and infection may also cause hyperglycemia. Diabetic acidosis can result over a period of hours or days. You had symptoms of hyperglycemia before coming into the hospital; they included excessive urination and thirst. You were tired, you lost weight, and you were dehydrated. Other signs and symptoms of hyperglycemia may include drowsiness, loss of appetite, blurred vision, abdominal pain, nausea, vomiting, and a fruity odor to your breath. To avoid hyperglycemia, follow your meal plan closely, test your blood glucose levels regularly, and report any consistently high levels. Call for an appointment with your physician or nurse practitioner when you have a fever or when a wound looks like it could be infected."

O (Outpatient/Inpatient Referrals): Sequential blood glucose monitoring: "The purpose of doing fingersticks with the glucometer before meals and at bedtime is to determine if the insulin and food you are taking are in the correct balance to control your blood glucose levels."

Provide local and national resources.

D (Diet): 1800-calorie ADA diet, no added sugar. Attach sample menu and exchange lists. Include significant others in teaching meal planning and following exchange lists.

Treatments

The patient, someone in his family, or another person must learn to use the glucometer, draw up and give insulin, and keep records of the patient's blood glucose levels and the amount of insulin administered. Including these items on your teaching plan would look like Box 4.3, listed under Treatments. Give the patient written instructions for how to use the glucometer and how to administer insulin. As you demonstrate how to check blood glucose levels and give an insulin injection, provide simple instructions for each step. Then ask the patient to give you a return demonstration, in which he tries to use the glucometer and give himself an insulin injection. Reassure and help him; he will be anxious at first.

Also, explain and demonstrate what the patient needs to do to care for his skin and feet. Again, have him give you a return demonstration. If the patient's nurse has already taught him these skills, check his understanding by asking him questions or watching him demonstrate them.

Health Knowledge of Disease

The patient needs to know the signs and symptoms of his disease and when it is time to call the physician or nurse practitioner. In this case, it is most important for the patient to know about hypoglycemia and hyperglycemia and what to do about these conditions when they occur. Review the signs and symptoms of hypoglycemia and hyperglycemia with the patient, and explain the circumstances most likely to precipitate symptoms. Again, consult Box 4.3 for an example of what your teaching plan might include.

Inpatient and Outpatient Referrals

Be prepared to explain any test or procedure in a sentence or two using nonmedical terminology. This particular patient is not scheduled for any blood tests in addition to his blood glucose levels. But be prepared to explain, as in Box 4.3, when, where, how, and why sequential blood glucose tests are needed as applicable to the situation.

There is no way to predict what other tests will be ordered, and you are not expected to memorize every single test. The more common tests will become familiar as your experiences and knowledge increase. An overview of some common tests, with normal values, was described in Chapter 2. There will always be references available on your unit for you to look up laboratory tests and procedures. You can also call the laboratory or department in which the test is being done and request patient information materials for the test or procedure.

It is helpful to give patients information on local and national resources concerning their health problems. The Internet is an excellent resource for locating addresses or phone numbers of agencies so that patients and their significant others have a place to start looking for more information if they are interested. For example, national diabetes resources include:

▶ American Diabetes Association, 1701 Beauregard Street, Alexandria, VA 22311; 1-800-DIABETES (1-800-342-2383); http://www.diabetes.org
▶ National Diabetes Education Program, http://www.ndep.nih.gov
▶ National Diabetes Information Clearinghouse, 1 Information Way, Bethesda, MD 20892-3560; http://diabetes.niddk.nih.gov

Once you know what the national organizations are, look in the phone book to determine whether there is a local branch of the organization. If there is, provide the patient or significant other with the appropriate phone number.

At this point in your planning process, you have no specific data about the patient's discharge. The physician or nurse practitioner will provide instructions for scheduling follow-up appointments and arranging for a home health-care agency, if necessary.

Diet

This patient has been prescribed an 1800-calorie ADA diet with no added sugar. You will need to teach him how to use a food exchange list. Fruits, breads, meats, fats, and milk products are grouped in lists. Exchange lists and sample menus may be obtained from the dietary department in the health-care agency. You can also obtain online information from the American Dietetic Association. The American Dietetic Association is the professional organization of dietitians, the same as the ANA is for nurses. The most up to date recommendations for nutrition of diabetics are available from this organization.

Plan to sit down with the patient to discuss the diet and the food lists. Ask him to plan his meals according to what he likes to eat, using the exchange lists. Plan to have significant others also listen to your instructions, especially the person who usually prepares the patient's meals.

The preceding discussion of the teaching plan includes details of teaching content and rationales. Your mini–teaching plan should be no more than one page long. It should provide an outline of what you will need to teach. Attach all relevant teaching materials you will be using. There is no need to rewrite and duplicate information found in the teaching materials and standardized care plans. The plan should contain the information listed in Box 4.3.

In summary, the METHOD daily teaching plan is a focused, individualized plan based on data from the concept care maps and general standardized teaching plans. You are expected to attach relevant teaching materials to the plan.

Developing Teaching Skills

To be an effective teacher, you must know not only what to teach but also how to teach it. You must assess the patient and significant others for learning readiness before trying to teach anything. For example, if the patient is highly anxious or in considerable pain, or if he is tired or hungry, you may try to teach him something; however, chances are that he will retain little of the information you provide, and he may become even more anxious.

To teach effectively, you will need to use basic principles of teaching and learning in adults and children, and you will need to use key adult learning principles, teaching strategies, and evaluation methods (Box 4.4). For further discussion of basic principles of learning and teaching strategies, refer to Chapter 11 in *Communication for Nurses: How to Prevent Harmful Events and Promote Patient Safety*.[3] Patient-safe communication is the foundation of the nurse-patient relationship. You must know how to use patient-safe communication strategies throughout the process of teaching.

Teaching plans focus on data from the concept care map and on general patient teaching information prioritized to address the most important problems first. Keep in mind that anxiety blocks communication and learning, and that even a calm patient can only absorb so much information at one time. When possible, ask the patient where he would like to start, and then be flexible. Bring your detailed, standardized care plans with you and refer to them if the patient asks questions you are not prepared to answer. Students are not expected to know every aspect of teaching about every health problem. As needed, refer questions to your clinical faculty, cover nurse, or the appropriate health-care personnel, such as the diabetes educator or dietitian in this example.

Box 4.4 ADULT LEARNING PRINCIPLES

Use these principles when teaching adult patients:
- Build on previous experiences.
- Focus on immediate concerns first.
- Adapt teaching to the patient's lifestyle.
- Make the patient an active participant.
- Determine learning readiness.
- Be realistic and stick to the basics.
- Take advantage of the teachable moment by incorporating teaching into your ongoing patient care.
- Reinforce all learning.
- Solicit feedback.

Knowledge-Based Teaching Strategies

Your teaching methods must coincide with the type of knowledge you are trying to convey. Use these techniques:
- *Cognitive knowledge (facts):* Give explanations and descriptions. Use books, pamphlets, films, programmed instruction, and computer programs.
- *Affective and cognitive knowledge (feelings and beliefs):* Use one-to-one discussions, group discussions, role-playing, and discovery to guide the patient in problem-solving situations that help him express feelings and use cognitive knowledge to solve problems.
- *Psychomotor knowledge (skills):* Use demonstrations accompanied by explanations.

Evaluation of Teaching: Did the Patient Learn?

To assess your patient's learning, use these techniques:
- *Cognitive knowledge:* Ask oral or written questions. Ask the patient to keep a diary or records of self-monitoring.
- *Affective knowledge:* Infer the patient's level of learning from how he responds to you, how he speaks about his illness and his treatments, and how he verbally expresses his feelings and values.
- *Psychomotor knowledge:* Ask the patient for a return demonstration.

CHAPTER 4 SUMMARY

The purpose of this chapter was to guide you in the development of step 4 of the concept care map. Step 4 involves prioritizing problems and then developing goals, outcomes, and nursing strategies for each diagnosis. Nursing strategies are developed to support patients physically and emotionally and to provide the services that patients cannot provide for themselves. Emotional support is as important as the physical care provided to patients.

Step 4 is based on thinking critically and synthesizing information from standardized care plans and the data available on the concept care map. Step 4 also involves developing a teaching plan for the patient and significant others. The components of the teaching plan for the day of care can be remembered using the acronym METHOD. These letters stand for the key elements of a teaching plan: medications, environment, treatments, health knowledge of disease, outpatient/inpatient referrals, and diet.

Carry your concept care map, goals, outcomes, strategies, and teaching plan in your pocket on the clinical unit. Also, bring the standardized care plans, clinical pathways (if available), medication cards or printouts, and relevant patient education materials as needed. In addition, bring the patient profile database with the fall-risk assessment and pressure ulcer risk assessment. What you need to bring to the clinical site is listed in Box 4.5.

Box 4.5   CHECKLIST: WHAT TO BRING TO THE CLINICAL AGENCY

1. Patient profile database
2. Concept care map based on patient profile database (steps 1–3)
3. Plan of Goals/Outcomes/Strategies (step 4)
4. Pressure ulcer risk assessment scale
5. Falls risk assessment scale
6. METHOD teaching plan
7. Patient education materials
8. Standardized care plans
9. Clinical pathways, if available
10. Printouts or medication cards for all drugs

LEARNING ACTIVITIES

To do these exercises, you will need access to books on medical-surgical nursing, nutrition, medications, diagnostic tests and procedures, and standardized care plans. One approach is to form a group ahead of time and have each person bring a specific reference to class, instead of having each student carry all of the references.

1. Work in groups of three or four students to develop step 4 goals, outcomes, and strategies for the patients in scenarios 2 and 3 in the learning activities for Chapter 3. Split up the diagnoses among the groups. Each group should write its goals, outcomes, and strategies on the board for critique by the entire class.

2. A representative of each group should state rationales for the strategies for the assigned diagnosis.

3. Develop METHOD teaching plans for the patients in Scenarios 2 and 3. Split up the components of the teaching plan (medications, environment, treatments, health knowledge of disease, outpatient/inpatient referrals, and diet) among the group. Write the teaching components on the board so the entire class can critique the content of the teaching plan.

4. A representative of each group should state the teaching methods that would be used to teach the information.

5. Using the diabetic patient in this chapter as an example, explain what you would say and do to assess his anxiety, show empathy, and use comfort touch and therapeutic humor.

REFERENCES

1. NANDA International. NANDA Nursing Diagnoses: Definitions and Classification, 10th ed. 2015–2017. Herdman TH, ed. Chichester, United Kingdom: Wiley-Blackwell; 2014.
2. *Nursing: Scope and Standards of Practice.* 2nd ed. Silver Spring, Md: American Nurses Association; 2010.
3. Schuster PM, Nykolyn L. *Communication for Nurses: How to Prevent Harmful Events and Promote Patient Safety.* Philadelphia, Pa: F.A. Davis; 2010.
4. Schuster PM. *Communication: The Key to the Therapeutic Relationship.* Philadelphia, Pa: F.A. Davis; 2000.
5. Huey R, et al. Discharge planning: Good planning means fewer hospitalizations for the chronically ill. *Nursing.* 1981; 81:11-20. (This is a classic seminal article.)

5

NURSING IMPLEMENTATION: USING CONCEPT CARE MAPS AS NURSING CARE PLANS AT THE HEALTH-CARE AGENCY

1. Describe strategies of clinical organizational strategies necessary for successful clinical performance.

2. Identify American Nurses Association (ANA) standards of professional nursing practice related to implementation and evaluation of nursing care plans in the health-care agency.

3. Describe how to update and modify a concept care map upon arrival at the clinical agency.

4. Relate how to use a concept care map during interactions with patients.

5. Describe how to evaluate patient responses to nursing strategies.

6. Describe how the concept care map can be used to facilitate communication among the student nurses, the clinical faculty, and the patient's staff nurse.

7. Use the concept care map to explain the relationship between medications and relevant clinical data before giving drugs.

8. Describe the development of concept care maps for use in outpatient settings.

The concept care map is used as an organizational tool for clinical data. One focus of this chapter is on organizational strategies to prioritize what must be done during a clinical day to implement the plan of care. This chapter also describes implementation and evaluation of nursing care using the concept care map.

Standard 5 of the ANA Standards of Professional Nursing Practice mandates that nurses take responsibility for the implementation of the patient's plan of care. This involves coordination of care delivery and use of strategies to promote health and a safe environment.[1] In the clinical setting, the concept care map becomes a dynamic working clinical patient care tool to assist you with organizing the data for the ongoing care of your patients.

Standard 6 of the ANA Standards of Professional Nursing Practice requires that nurses take responsibility for evaluating patients' progress toward attaining their outcomes and goals.[1] This is accomplished by identifying patient responses to prescribed strategies, which is step 5 of completing the concept care map. You must discipline yourself to focus carefully on and evaluate patient responses to each prescribed strategy, and you must record these responses on the concept care map. In addition, you must also determine the patient's viewpoint regarding his or her progress toward the outcome objectives.

The nurse revises the plan of care based on evaluations, reorders priorities, and establishes new goals, outcomes, and treatment strategies as needed to maximize the patient's health capabilities.[1] Therefore, you must be able to update the concept care map to account for dynamic changes that regularly occur in clinical settings. You will face many challenges throughout a clinical day; nothing ever goes exactly as planned!

Arrival at the Inpatient Unit: Getting Organized

Getting organized is crucial for successful clinical performance. When you arrive at the clinical unit, you must obtain the latest data on medications, IV fluids, and treatments, along with a patient status report. Write updates directly on your concept care map "sloppy copy." Put new data on the "sloppy copy" under the appropriate diagnoses. Do not use a separate sheet of paper for the updates, because a separate sheet of paper could easily get lost. Use a red pen so you and your clinical faculty can quickly see your revisions. A prioritized list of all the activities you must complete to update your plan of care is shown in Box 5.1.

Check Medication Records

Check for changes in the patient's medications by reviewing medication records for routine and as-needed (prn) drugs. Update your concept care map by adding, deleting, or revising drugs. Write the times at which medications should be administered on the front of the map in red ink. Highlight medications so you can find them easily on the concept care map. Write down on the concept care map what time the patient last received a prn pain medication as well as the name of the drug. If you are not familiar with any of the drugs the patient is receiving, before giving the medications look them up in a drug reference book, or call the pharmacy to obtain information.

Check IV Administration Records

Check for changes in the patient's IV records. Record the current fluid being administered and the rate of administration on the concept care map diagram in the appropriate nursing diagnosis box. Highlight the intravenous fluid and rate of administration. Also note and highlight admixtures and length of infusion time.

Box 5.1	WHAT TO DO WHEN YOU ARRIVE AT THE UNIT

1. Check the patient's medication record.
2. Check the patient's IV administration record.
3. Check the patient's treatments.
4. Check the patient's laboratory data.
5. Obtain a patient report from the off-going shift.

Check Treatments

Check for updates in the patient's treatments, and write these on the concept care map in the appropriate nursing diagnosis box. If the information does not fit in any of the diagnostic boxes that appear on the map, make a new diagnosis box. If you are not sure where the new information goes, place it in a box labeled "I don't know how this fits with the problems" and check with your clinical faculty.

Check Laboratory Data

Check the records for laboratory tests and diagnostic procedures that were ordered from the time you left the unit. Find out which laboratory tests and procedures were completed and which reports are pending. For completed laboratory tests and procedures, find the reports and write the results on your concept care map in the appropriate diagnostic categories. For pending laboratory results, write in the name of the test and place a blank next to it so you will know to fill in the result when it becomes available. Typically, the daily morning blood work is drawn between 5 and 6 a.m., and laboratory reports come back to the units early. You must have the latest information on laboratory data before administering many of the patient's drugs. For example, if you need to give Lanoxin (digoxin) and Lasix (furosemide), you will first need to know the most recent potassium value.

It is also crucial to analyze blood samples that are related to medications, because side effects of medications are often detected through analysis of blood samples. In this example, Lasix causes potassium to be lost in the urine, and hypokalemia may result.

Obtain Information from the Previous Shift

There is always an end-of-shift summary report for each patient. It is crucial that you obtain a report of the patient's recent health status. Change-of-shift reports may take many different forms, including:

- A verbal report, with all oncoming nursing staff taking notes on all patients
- Tape-recorded reports
- Written reports
- Verbal one-on-one reports between the nurse who is leaving and the nurse who is starting to deliver care to a particular group of patients

Write the information you obtain from the change-of-shift report in the appropriate nursing diagnosis boxes on your map. If necessary, make a new box if the data suggests a new nursing diagnosis. If you do not know where new information belongs on your map, put it in the box labeled "I don't know how this fits with the problems" and check with your clinical faculty.

In short, as soon as you get to the health-care agency, start collecting data to update your concept care map sloppy copy. Obtain data from medication records, IV records, treatments, laboratory data, and staff nurses. Look at the laboratory data that were recently collected and note any laboratory data that are pending. Medications are usually the priority; many (such as insulin and Lasix) must be given on time. It is also important to give pain medications on time. Always check medications first, because you may need to give a medication before doing anything else.

The nurses at the end of their shift will be busy finishing their documentation and preparing their reports for the oncoming shift. This is not a good time to ask them questions. The outgoing nurses will give you and the oncoming nurses shift reports as scheduled, when they have completed their work. After the shift report, you may ask them additional questions before they leave.

Clinical Preconference

For many students, a clinical preconference is held early in the clinical day, after the change-of-shift report. The purpose of the preconference is for clinical faculty to meet with students and review the accuracy of the concept care map. By looking at your concept care map, your clinical faculty will be able to see very quickly if you have collected, correctly analyzed, categorized, and prioritized data. Goals, outcomes, and strategies are reviewed quickly. Succinct lists on a concept care map facilitate a rapid evaluation of the plan of care.

You must be prepared to address questions concerning your plan of care. This includes assessment data, nursing and medical diagnoses, goals, outcomes, strategies, and rationales. Your faculty may prefer that you write out rationales for all strategies you plan to implement. After the preconference, keep the concept care map in your pocket to guide you throughout the day.

Updating Assessments, Reporting Findings, and Giving Medications

After determining your initial priorities and completing your preconference, you will most likely need to accomplish several more specific tasks (Box 5.2). These tasks include patient assessment, reporting the findings of your assessment, and preparing to give medications.

Patient Assessment and Evaluation

If the patient is sleeping, wake him to do your first assessment of the clinical day. If you are like many beginning students, you may not want to disturb the patient's sleep. It is critical, however, that you have the assessment data you need to make sound clinical judgments. In fact, it is possible that the patient is not sleeping but is comatose, and you would not know that unless you attempted to awaken him. A diabetic patient could be unconscious from hypoglycemia. It is a professional standard of care that assessments are done on each patient early at the start of each shift. Write your findings in the evaluation column of your care plan, shown in Figure 5.1. The recorded notes of patient responses fall under step 5 of the concept care map. These notes will be the basis of documentation that will be explained in Chapter 7.

Start your assessments by performing the key assessments first. If your patient needs to go for a test, or your clinical faculty or his doctor or nurse come in to see the patient, you will be able to report your findings. All health-care providers will want to know the key assessments, so always do the key assessments first; they are the most

---

Box 5.2   WHAT TO DO AFTER UPDATING THE CARE PLAN

1. Perform patient assessment.
2. Report assessment data to patient's assigned staff nurse.
3. Report assessment data to clinical faculty.
4. Locate medications.
5. Meet faculty in medication area to prepare for drug administration (if applicable).

---

important. The key assessments for the patient newly diagnosed with diabetes were signs and symptoms of hypoglycemia and hyperglycemia, blood glucose value, food intake, and vital signs. The key assessments that you must do first are going to be different for each patient. It is important to note that the patient response is to be recorded, not the fact that you did the prescribed strategy. The recorded notes of patient responses are the fifth step of the concept care map shown in Figure 5.1.

Reporting Assessment Data

After you have done your assessment and evaluation and have taken notes, you need to quickly find your patient's assigned staff nurse, introduce yourself if necessary, and report your assessment findings. If you see your clinical faculty before you see the patient's nurse, report your findings to the clinical faculty. Assessment and patient evaluation involves critical information that both your faculty and patient's assigned staff nurse want to know as soon as possible, during the first hour of the shift.

Once the patient's immediate needs are met, you need to review with the patient's assigned staff nurse what you will and will not be doing for patient care. You may need to say, "I don't know how to do the dressing change yet" or "I haven't learned to use the glucometer." The staff nurse is responsible for doing what you have not yet learned to do, so you must be very clear about what you can do and what she will need to do.

Problem # _____1_____ : Imbalanced Nutrition: Less than body requirements
General Goal: To improve the patient's nutritional status

Predicted Behavioral Outcome Objective (s): The patient will…maintain his blood glucose between 80 and 120 mg/dl by eating his 1800-calorie ADA diet and administering insulin injections as scheduled…on the day of care.

Nursing Strategies	Patient Responses
1. Assess abdomen: bowel sounds, tenderness, distention, BMs	1. BS all quads, nontender, nondistended, no BM
2. Assess blood glucose with glucometer at 0800 and 1100	2. 60 at 7:30, 100 at 11:30
3. Assess S/S of hypoglycemia and hyperglycemia	3. 7:45, clammy/sweaty, dizzy, hungry
4. Monitor appetite–1800 cal ADA, no sugar added	4. Ate 90% breakfast, 50% lunch
5. Measure fluid intake and output	5. I=400, 350, 200 0=250, 225, 300
6. Administer insulin on time	6. 8:00 insulin held, Dr. notified, continue glucometer measurements and call for further orders after each BS
7. Check for additional blood work	7. K=3.8
8. Monitor patient for orthostatic hypotension and weakness	8. Steady while standing and walking BP 124/60 standing
9. Ambulate carefully to avoid falls	9. Able to walk without assistance to BR

Evaluation: Summarize patient progress toward outcome objectives: Need to continue to carefully monitor for hypoglycemia and hyperglycemia because diet, insulin, and blood sugar still not coordinated, is stronger and is cautious with movement.

Problem # _____2_____ : Anxiety
General Goal: Decrease anxiety

Predicted Behavioral Outcome Objective (s): The patient will…verbalize concerns about his disease and the changes that must be made in his lifestyle…on the day of care.

Nursing Strategies	Patient Responses
1. Assess current level of anxiety	1. Appeared anxious during hypoglycemic episode
2. Use empathy	2. Verbalized concerns about disease
3. Use therapeutic touch	3. Accepted touch, eased anxiety
4. Use therapeutic humor	4. Responded by smiling, eased anxiety

Evaluation: Summarize patient progress toward outcome objectives: Patient stated he was concerned about learning how to give his own injections and how to prepare meals. Communication techniques effective in gaining cooperation and mutual goal setting, and helped to control anxiety by verbalization of concerns.

Problem # _____3_____ : Deficient knowledge
General Goal: Increase knowledge

Predicted Behavioral Outcome Objective (s): The patient will…decide in collaboration with the nurse what aspects of diabetic teaching protocol he would like to focus on during… the day of care.

Nursing Strategies	Patient Responses
1. Assess current level of knowledge and establish what the patient most wants to learn about during the day of care	1. Wants to know about hypoglycemia, glucometer monitoring, and insulin injections
2. Assess resources available for teaching, such as diabetic educator, dietitian, programs, or movies	2. Diabetes educator visited and will start classes at outpatient clinic when discharged
3. See teaching plan for: –what diabetes is and how it affects health (signs and symptoms) –Medications –Diet –Skin care –Exercise/activity	3. Focused on signs and symptoms, use of glucometer, drawing up insulin, see teaching plan for evaluation of teaching

Evaluation: Summarize patient progress toward outcome objectives: Needs continued practice to use glucometer. Did not need insulin this shift so could not practice self-administration. Did correctly draw up the medication. Can state the signs of hypoglycemia and hyperglycemia. Review of menus not done due to lack of time.

● Figure 5.1   Steps 4 and 5 of the concept care map.

Problem #____4____: Ineffective Peripheral Tissue Perfusion General Goal: Maintain optimal tissue perfusion and circulation	
Predicted Behavioral Outcome Objective (s): The patient will...have vital signs remaining close to normal, no skin breakdown, moves safely from bed to chair...on the day of care.	
Nursing Strategies	Patient Responses
1. Assess vital signs 2. Assess peripheral pulses and capillary refill 3. Assess skin for pressure sore 4. Give valsartan, assess BP/P prior to administrations 5. ROM extremities q2h if in bed 6. Walk w/assistance 7. Chair x 2	1. 0800=140/85 98.6-20 1230=128/74 98.4-72-18 2. 3+ pedals, capillary refill <3 sec 3. No redness or broken areas 4. 0900 BP 148/84, p=82 Gave valsartan 5. Does active ROM q2h while in bed and in chair 6. Walked to BR without assistance 7. 0900 sat in chair 60 min, 1330 sat in chair 60 min
Evaluation: Summarize patient progress toward outcome objectives: BP controlled with medication, no orthostatic hypotension, strength improving, ambulating well, no skin breakdown	

Problem #____5____: Impaired Physical Mobility General Goal: Prevent complications of immobility, prevent falls	
Predicted Behavioral Outcome Objective (s): The patient will...ambulate to chair and walk without steady gait, otherwise does range of motion exercises...on the day of care.	
Nursing Strategies	Patient Responses
1. Covered under Nutrition and Altered tissue perfusion	
Evaluation: Summarize patient progress toward outcome objectives: Covered under nutrition and altered tissue perfusion	

Problem #____6____: Impaired Urinary Elimination General Goal: Mantain normal urinary elimination	
Predicted Behavioral Outcome Objective (s): The patient will...have intake and ouput approaching normal values, no polyuria...on the day of care.	
Nursing Strategies	Patient Responses
1. Covered under Nutrition	
Evaluation: Summarize patient progress toward outcome objectives: No polyuria, output listed above.	

● Figure 5.1 Continued

She may review the daily plan of care with you, emphasizing from her viewpoint the important aspects of care that must be done.

Communication must flow openly between you, the faculty, and the patient's staff nurse. Any time you find abnormalities in any of your patient's assessment data (be sure to report abnormal key assessment data first), interrupt the staff nurse or your clinical faculty to report abnormalities. The key words here are *interrupt* and *any abnormalities*. Abnormalities include anything not within normal parameters; for example, a blood pressure of 150/92 is not within normal parameters. Many students hesitate to interrupt when the faculty or staff nurses look busy. Get the

attention of one or the other no matter how busy they might appear. Abnormal assessment data mean the patient could be in trouble, and the staff nurse and clinical faculty have the knowledge to make a clinical judgment about what is an imminent danger and what can wait until later. Each of these nurses will want to personally assess and evaluate the patient's responses, to validate your findings.

Even if you find and interrupt your clinical faculty and she tells you that she cannot come to the patient's bedside immediately, she will tell you to find the patient's assigned staff nurse or the charge nurse. She will check on you and your patient as soon as possible. If the staff nurse and clinical faculty are both too busy, they will refer you to yet another nurse.

Finding Medications

After the assessment and report phase, the next step is to find all your medications for the shift. You have already checked the medication administration record and made updates. Now you actually have to find the drugs. Check to make sure all the pills, injections, liquids, eye drops, inhalants, IV medications, and other required items are on the unit. Medications may be in a medication cart or refrigerator, or at the bedside. Some may come from a computerized dispenser. Carefully check all currently available drugs. For a drug that is not normally kept on the unit, you may need to follow hospital policy to obtain it. To do so, you may need to call the pharmacy, fax an order, or go to the pharmacy to pick up the drug. Once you have found all your patient's medications, meet your clinical faculty in the medication area early in the shift to discuss administration.

The concept care map is particularly useful as you and your clinical faculty analyze relationships between the patient's laboratory data, physical assessment data, and medications. For example, the discussion of the relationship between insulin, blood glucose level, and appetite is facilitated because all of these items are in the same diagnostic box. Likewise, a discussion of the need to assess the patient's blood pressure before giving the antihypertensive drug valsartan (Diovan) is facilitated because they are in the same box. When you see drugs, laboratory work, and physical assessment data under the same diagnosis, identify the significant relationships between data. You will soon realize that you must know the blood glucose level to decide whether or not to give the patient his insulin. If his blood glucose level is too low, you could harm the patient by giving the drug.

Using The Concept Care Map to Facilitate Communication

The concept care map is a bridge that facilitates communication between you and your clinical faculty. As clinical faculty make bedside rounds, the concept care map allows you to easily discuss the patient's progress toward or away from goals and outcomes. As a result of your discussion, you can make notes and revisions on the concept care map or nursing strategy lists.

Bedside Communication

Bedside rounds occur periodically throughout the day. Assessment data can be validated by your faculty or staff nurse or corrected if inaccurate, and concept care maps can be updated as a result of rounds. Faculty comments should appear on your map in a distinct color, such as purple or green, so that these comments are easily visible. Faculty may make written notations instructing you to continue to assess certain aspects of care, to try specific strategies, or to illustrate the finer aspects of the interrelationships of care. Because concept care maps show a comprehensive picture of the patient, they facilitate a thorough discussion between you and your faculty.

For example, the clinical faculty might walk into the room and say, "Let's see your diagram on the sloppy copy, patient objectives, and strategy lists." The faculty may then proceed to ask questions such as "How is he eating? What's his last blood glucose? Any signs of hypoglycemia? How much is he urinating? How's his blood pressure and pulse? What have you covered so far in your teaching?" These questions can be addressed by reviewing the updated concept care map.

Reporting Off the Unit

You are responsible to report to the patient's assigned staff nurse before going on breaks and before going home. Never leave a unit without giving a report to the patient's assigned staff nurse. Focus the report on the key areas of assessment that are most crucial to the care of the patient, located centrally on the diagram under the reason for admission to the health-care facility. If anything else is abnormal, be sure to tell the staff nurse. Get out your concept care map and use it to remind yourself of what you need to say. For example, as you go to lunch at 11:40 a.m., you tell the staff nurse, "He hasn't had any more signs of hypoglycemia, and the 11:30 fingerstick was 100. He did it himself, but still can't remember the exact procedure without help. The doctor wants to be notified about the glucose. The patient's eating in bed right now. Everything else is fine."

Implementation for the Diabetic Patient

The diabetic patient who appeared in earlier chapters will help to illustrate the process of organizing, implementing, and evaluating patient care. Start by reviewing the concept care map shown in Figure 5.2. It has been updated after a review of patient records and the shift report. On the concept care map diagram, medications are highlighted to make them more prominent.

Assessment

First, you must do a head-to-toe physical assessment of the patient. Focus on assessing what you have determined to be essential key assessments, which are written in the center box on your concept care map under the patient's reason for needing health care. A head-to-toe assessment is the most important way to obtain

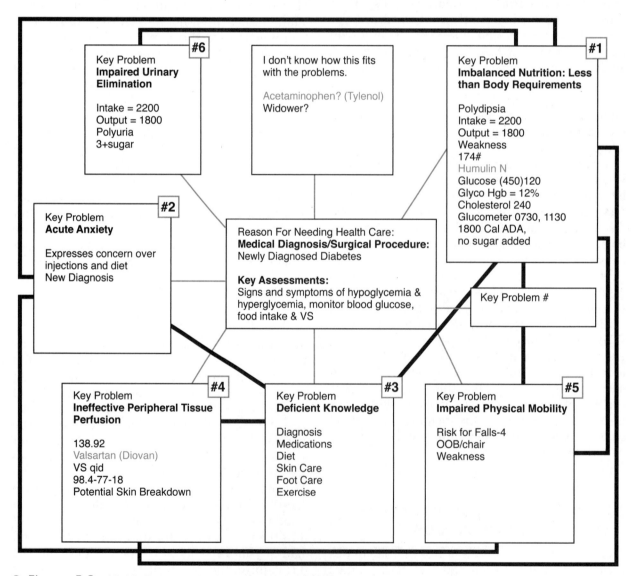

Figure 5.2   Highlight your patient's medications on the diagram.

baseline data at the start of the shift. You must be thorough. If you check a patient's lungs, check all lung fields. Student nurses sometimes hesitate to "disturb" a patient to do a complete assessment. The patient may be in pain, he may be immobilized for any number of reasons, or he may simply be asleep. If necessary, get an assistant to hold the patient up while you assess all lung fields and perform the rest of your assessment. Physical assessments are done at least once a shift, more often if the patient's acuity level makes them necessary.

For the diabetic patient, you should ask the patient about signs and symptoms of hypoglycemia and hyperglycemia, obtain results of his blood glucose test, and ask about food intake. As you greet the patient with a handshake, start with a general question, such as "How are you doing this morning?" Listen carefully to see if the patient says anything that could suggest a problem.

Consider this scenario: He keeps hold of your hand and says that he feels sweaty and light-headed this morning. He is responding to your touch by holding onto you. You ask if he is hungry. He says yes. You ask if he is feeling numb anywhere. He says no. You say, "I'll check your blood sugar and see what it is." You next check his blood glucose level using the glucometer and find it to be 60. You also find that his blood pressure is 140/85, his pulse is 86, and his respirations are 20. Quickly write the blood glucose level and vital signs on the care plan so you don't forget them.

From these data, you conclude that the patient is hypoglycemic but stable. You ask if he can eat his breakfast and he says yes. You get the tray, open some orange juice for him, and watch while he drinks it. If the tray is not yet available, you can get him orange juice and crackers. Then you immediately report what happened to the patient's staff nurse and your clinical faculty. Recount the patient's report of symptoms, the blood glucose level, the vital signs, and what you did about the patient's problem.

Suppose you do not know how to use the glucometer. In that case, you would quickly take the patient's blood pressure, pulse, and respirations, and conclude that he is probably hypoglycemic but has stable vital signs. Immediately ask your faculty or the patient's staff nurse to check his blood glucose level. Tell the staff nurse you have not yet learned to use the glucometer, and ask her to do it. You will have the staff nurse's immediate, undivided attention if you tell her the patient is having a hypoglycemic reaction. This problem needs immediate attention in order to intervene before it gets any worse.

Establish Mutual Goals

After performing your assessment, you must negotiate with the patient to establish mutual goals, expected outcomes, and a schedule of activities. Use the list of goals, outcomes, and strategies that you already constructed and, in very simple terms, review with the patient what needs to be done. Discuss each of the problems and listen carefully to what the patient believes should be the goals and outcomes of care for the day.

For example, you know that the patient needs to do morning care, to get up safely into a chair, to learn about self-care and diabetes, and especially to learn what to do about hypoglycemic reactions. As you review these activites with the patient, use empathy and humor to establish a professional nurse-patient relationship. By using communication strategies, you will be better able to find out what the patient is thinking. For instance, you may discover that he is especially concerned about fluctuations in his blood glucose levels and regulation of insulin with his meals. Of course, you will have things that you consider to be important. You will want to discuss his weakness and his risk of falling. Tell him to be cautious when getting up, and explain that you want to be present when he does get up so you can check his blood pressure. List the major items the patient needs to learn for self-care, and let the patient select which aspects of teaching he wants to start with. This portion of the day is about establishing agreements and goals. A successful outcome of your conversation with him thus far would be for him to say that he will not get out of bed without calling you, and that he wants to learn how to check his blood glucose after morning care. The goals, outcomes, and strategies you established in the plan of care will guide your discussions with the patient in the morning and throughout the day.

Implementing and Evaluating Care

Make sure you do everything you said you were going to do on your plan of care. Some students prefer to check off each item on the list of strategies as they do them so they do not forget to do anything. Your clinical faculty and the patient's staff nurse will be expecting you to either carry out each nursing strategy you listed in step 4 or report that it could not get done in a timely manner. For example, say you write that the patient is to do range-of-motion exercises every 2 hours. You are responsible for checking every 2 hours and for reminding the patient to do these exercises if he forgets. Failure to carry out all established strategies as planned and in a timely manner is negligent, and is considered malpractice. Therefore, make sure you keep your faculty informed, no matter how busy they may appear.

As you perform interventions, evaluate the patient's responses to assess his progress toward expected outcomes throughout the day. Record these responses in a different color ink in the column across from your intervention list (see Fig. 5.1).

Step 5 includes writing down an evaluation summary of the patient's progress toward the outcome objectives. This summary includes your clinical judgments. Carefully consider the effectiveness of your strategies in bringing about the expected patient outcomes. If your strategies are not working and the patient is not progressing as anticipated, your clinical faculty and the patient's assigned staff nurse are there to help you consider other strategies and to make revisions in the concept care map.

Evaluate the patient's verbal and nonverbal behaviors regarding each item on the strategy list throughout the day. Carefully consider physical assessment data. Take notes as you go along. You will probably not be doing the strategies in the order you have written them on the nursing strategy "to do" lists, but that is fine. Since strategies are not done in order, you should check off each item as you do it, to keep track of what has been done.

Evaluation of the Teaching Plan

Your teaching plan must be evaluated like your basic care plan (see Box 4.3 in Chapter 4 to review the teaching plan). Focus on teaching methods, responses of the patient or significant others to teaching, and knowledge gained by the patient (Box 5.3). Also note what should be taught and what should be reinforced by the patient's next nurse to ensure continuity of care.

Other Outcomes to Review

Evaluate the patient's outcomes against standardized care plans and clinical paths. As you evaluate, you learn to predict expected patient responses and to judge how your patient compares to the expected outcomes for the "typical" patient. Nurses use standardized plans and clinical paths to double check that everything that was supposed to be done was done. In addition, falls and skin assessments with expected outcomes must be evaluated.

Inpatient Versus Outpatient Settings

An obvious difference between inpatient and outpatient units is the acuity level of the patients. Although patients are typically healthier in outpatient settings, you will still need to perform careful assessments, make nursing diagnoses, establish outcomes, carry out the nursing strategies, and evaluate patient responses. It is not possible to complete an individualized care plan ahead of time for an outpatient. Standardized plans of care and clinical pathways are used as guides for outpatient care. Preparation for an outpatient visit involves reviewing the typical procedures and plans of care that are used in the outpatient setting.

For example, in an endoscopy department, you would review the department's endoscopy procedure flow sheets, preprocedure and postprocedure orders, standardized discharge instructions, and conscious sedation flow sheets. You could use a medical-surgical textbook to review general symptoms and typical diseases diagnosed using endoscopy procedures. You also must be aware of possible complications during and after the procedure, and carefully monitor patients throughout their time in the department.

Box 5.3   EVALUATION OF TEACHING PLAN AND PATIENT LEARNING

Teaching Techniques
  Evaluation: Used discussion, question and answers, and demonstrations.

M (Medications)
  Evaluation: Discussed each medication. Patient knew the purpose of each drug. Was checking his own blood pressure each week at home using a cuff he bought at the drugstore. Needs to review side effects and precautions of insulin and valsartan. Received printed drug information.

E (Environment)
  Evaluation: Patient lives next door to his son, who checks on him daily and will help with meals, medication administration, getting to appointments, and so on. Verbalizes activity restrictions in the hospital.

T (Treatments)
  Evaluation: Glucometer demonstrated, and patient did his own fingerstick.

Received printed instructions for operating machine. Insulin not given, but patient drew up practice dose without assistance.

H (Health Knowledge of Disease)
  Evaluation: Verbalizes signs and symptoms of hypoglycemia and hyperglycemia. States what to do to avoid hypoglycemia and hyperglycemia. Relates symptoms experienced in a.m. to signs and symptoms of hypoglycemia.

O (Outpatient/Inpatient Referrals)
  Evaluation: States purpose of doing finger-sticks and sequential monitoring. Received information for national and regional resources.

D (Diet)
  Evaluation: Patient was tired and needed a rest, so unable to finish diet teaching. Information given to nurse who will be doing evening care. Planning to teach diet with son in attendance.

After reviewing these materials, it would be possible for you to make predictions about possible key nursing diagnoses and develop a concept care map that might look like Figure 5.3.

Once you and the patient arrive on the endoscopy outpatient unit, you must gather assessment data. For example, Figure 5.4 illustrates information gathered from a 47-year-old woman before she had an endoscopy procedure in the outpatient department.

During the procedure, the patient's blood pressure, pulses, respirations, pulse oximetry, and level of consciousness will be carefully monitored. She will receive drugs for sedation and pain. After the procedure, the nurse will perform a head-to-toe assessment, with special consideration for the gastrointestinal system and elimination. The nurse will be sure the following outcomes are attained before discharge:

- Stable vital signs
- Patent airway
- Intact gag reflex
- No nausea, vomiting, and dizziness
- Oral fluids tolerated
- Able to ambulate
- Able to void
- Comfortable pain level
- Understands home-going instructions

The pace of care in outpatient settings is very rapid. The nurses rapidly and continually assess, diagnose, plan, implement, and evaluate as the patient responds to the phases of the procedure and recovers from conscious sedation.

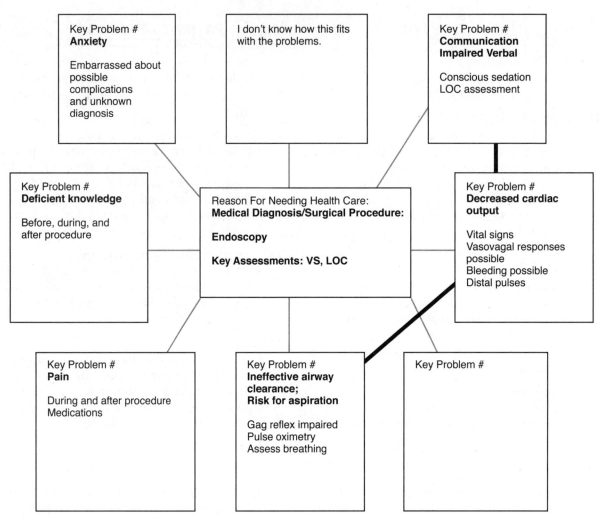

● Figure 5.3   Endoscopy procedure concept care map.

Reason for procedure	*Recheck site where large polyp was removed and patient had large blood loss during removal procedure*
Medical diagnosis	*Polyps*
Procedure	*Colonoscopy with possible biopsy, polypectomy, or both*
IV	*No. 18 angiocatheter with 1000 cc 0.9% normal saline solution in right antecubital space*
Vital signs	*BP = 133/70* *T = 95.8°F* *P = 68* *R = 20*
Height and weight	*5'5"* *120 lb*
Review of systems	*WNL all systems* *SaO$_2$ 99%*
Psychosocial-cultural assessment	*Catholic* *Married* *Anthem insurance* *Manager of a credit union* *During head-to-toe assessment, patient said she was nervous and afraid because of bad experience with bleeding when polyp was removed during the last procedure. Said she wanted to be completely knocked out for the procedure. Wanted a guarantee that she would not bleed like last time. Was visibly shaking.*

● Figure 5.4   Patient data for endoscopy procedure.

CHAPTER 5 SUMMARY

The focus of this chapter is organizational strategies to promote the safest, most efficient, and most productive clinical day. The chapter also focuses on using concept care maps as tools for clinical organization. Concept care maps are useful for organizing data in both inpatient and outpatient settings.

Concept care maps are used to organize and update patient assessment information, medications, IV fluids, treatments, and laboratory data when you arrive at the clinical unit. They are used to guide your patient assessments and evaluation of patient responses. They can be used to facilitate communication at the patient's bedside, in the medication area, and when you leave the unit for a break or at the end of the clinical day.

Step 5 of the concept care map is to take notes on patient responses to nursing strategies, evaluate outcomes, and record an evaluative summary of the patient's progress toward outcome objectives. You must evaluate the patient's verbal and nonverbal behaviors, gather physical assessment data, and write notes in the patient response to nursing strategies column of the nursing concept care map. These notes are the basis of documentation, which will be the focus of Chapter 7.

LEARNING ACTIVITIES

1. Preconference activity: Students should make comparisons with other students regarding medical and nursing diagnoses, concept care map diagrams, goals, objectives, and nursing strategy lists. For example, if one student has a postoperative patient with a hip replacement and another student has a patient with a knee replacement, these students should compare concept care maps. The purpose of this exercise is to find similarities common to postoperative orthopedic patients and to become cognizant of individual differences among patients and treatment plans.

2. Devise, implement, and evaluate a plan of care on a real patient assignment in an inpatient or outpatient setting.

3. Class exercise: The purpose of this exercise is to compare step 5 patient responses in patients with similar diagnoses. Students should bring a completed concept care map to class. Students assigned patients with similar diagnoses should form groups and review patient responses to nursing strategies. It should become apparent that, although patients may have similar medical and nursing diagnoses, the verbal and nonverbal responses listed under step 5 are unique, and progress toward outcomes varies from patient to patient.

4. Compare and contrast the concept care map developed for a diabetic inpatient with the concept care map developed for an outpatient undergoing endoscopy.

REFERENCE

1. *Nursing: Scope and Standards of Practice.* 2nd ed Silver Spring, Md: American Nurses Association; 2010.

6

MAPPING PSYCHOSOCIAL AND CULTURAL PROBLEMS

OBJECTIVES

1. Identify crucial psychosocial and cultural characteristics to assess.

2. Describe how to perform the psychosocial and cultural assessment.

3. Integrate psychosocial and cultural diagnoses into the concept care map.

4. Develop goals, outcomes, and strategies for psychosocial and cultural diagnoses.

5. Record the patient's psychosocial and cultural responses.

6. Analyze relationships among psychosocial, cultural, and physical diagnoses.

7. Describe the importance of patient-safe communication strategies to prevent harmful events in health-care settings.

The purpose of this chapter is to expand on the assessment, diagnosis planning, implementation, and evaluation of psychosocial-cultural problems. The patient profile database used in chapter 2 focused on the collection of relevant data the night before clinical or the day of clinical, primarily from patient records, a brief introduction to the patient and a brief discussion with the patient's staff nurse. Most of the information in patient records is primarily physical data, with only a small amount of psychosocial and cultural data. Therefore, you will need to communicate with patients directly to adequately assess their psychosocial and cultural problems.

You need time to communicate with patients to establish effective nurse-patient relationships with them. You also need to use patient-safe communication strategies to identify and manage psychosocial and cultural problems; make appropriate psychosocial and cultural nursing diagnoses; develop appropriate goals, outcomes, and strategies; and evaluate patient responses. This chapter will focus on how to develop concept care maps for psychosocial and cultural problems and the importance of patient-safe communication strategies in preventing harmful events.

Psychosocial, Cultural, and Developmental Assessment

Fundamental to the entire care planning and delivery process is your ability to communicate with high level competence and to form professional nurse-patient relationships, as well as communicate with members of the health-care team. Communication errors are the root cause of 70% of sentinel events in health-care settings.[1] The critical connection between communication and patient safety is that every aspect of patient care depends on available information that has been communicated between patients and health-care providers.[2] The transformational model of communication in Figure 6.1 delineates the complexity of communication dependent on context and depicts communication risk factors and patient-safe communication strategies to reduce miscommunications.

The psychosocial and cultural assessment of the patient and family is a critical assessment that requires high level communication competence. This assessment is also important prior to patient teaching that is needed for patients and families to attain health-care literacy. Assessing a patient's psychosocial and cultural status is not the same as taking a history and performing a physical examination. In contrast to the history and the physical, the psychosocial and cultural assessment is not based on direct questioning or interviewing.

Your objective is to develop rapport and a collaborative relationship with your patients. Nurses

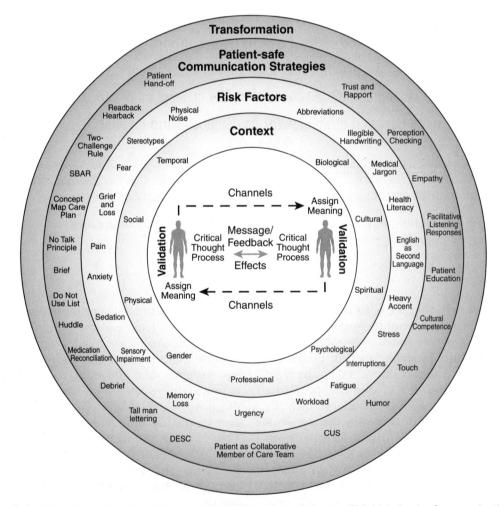

● Figure 6.1   Transformational model of communication. (From Schuster PM, Nykolyn L. *Communication for Nurses: How to Prevent Harmful Events and Promote Patient Safety*. Philadelphia, Pa: F.A. Davis; 2010.)

must be able to have a comfortable conversation with a patient. The purpose of developing rapport is to help the patient relax enough to verbalize psychosocial and cultural concerns whenever they arise. Thus, the psychosocial and cultural assessment is integrated into and continues throughout basic patient care. You may have a number of physical goals to attain with your patient, such as improving skin integrity, decreasing pain, increasing cardiac output, improving gas exchange, and improving nutrition. As you work to attain these goals, you will need to work simultaneously on assessment, diagnosis, and management of the patient's psychosocial and cultural problems.

Simultaneous assessment, diagnosis, and management of problems can be a difficult process to internalize and perform. But you and your patient are both assessing and responding to each other minute-to-minute. As a professional nurse, your assessments and responses must be finely tuned to move the patient toward a healthier physical, psychological, and sociocultural state (or a peaceful death), even while you are in the process of gathering data. You must learn the components of the psychosocial and cultural assessment very well so you know what to assess when interacting with your patients. You must learn appropriate verbal and nonverbal psychosocial and cultural responses, which have been described as *patient-safe communication strategies* by Schuster and Nykolyn.[2] Nurses strive to produce accurate messages through deliberate choice of patient-safe communication strategies while they monitor and respond to the emotions and reactions of patients and family members.[2] This communication process is depicted in Figure 6.2. For a comprehensive discussion of patient safety and patient-safe communication strategies, read Schuster and Nykolyn's *Communication for Nurses: How to Prevent Harmful Events and Promote Patient Safety.*

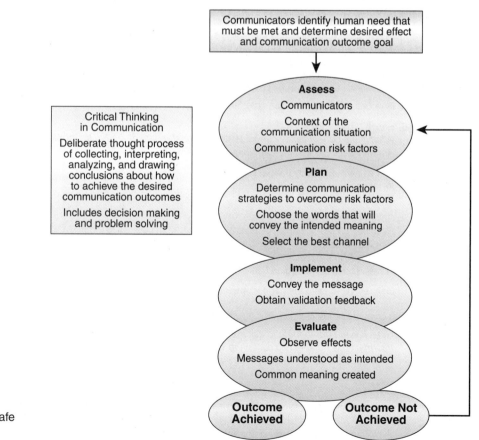

● Figure 6.2 Patient-safe communication process.

Assessment of Psychosocial and Cultural Problems

The psychosocial and cultural assessment tool that appears in Figure 6.3 has been developed as a guide for student nurses to use during clinical interactions with patients. The purpose of this assessment tool is to serve as a general critical-thinking guide for assessing psychosocial and cultural problems. These problems can be very complex, perhaps even more complex than physical problems. There are numerous psychosocial and cultural nursing diagnoses, and it helps to have a foundational assessment tool as a general guideline. Therefore, the purpose of this assessment tool is to give you a starting point for collecting psychosocial and cultural data. It contains eight important components: the patient's current emotional state, life experiences, family, growth and development issues, relations with health-care providers, self-concept, culture, and gender. Each section below is numbered to correspond with the tool in Figure 6.3.

Clinical Judgment_____

♦ 1. Emotional State
   Mood
   Body language
   Facial

♦ 2. Patient's Life Experience
   What are previous experiences with health care?

♦ 3. Family
   What is the mood of family members you meet?
   Are family members supportive?

♦ 4. Growth and Development–**Intimacy vs. Isolation**–Form an intimate bond with another person, growing independent of parents and managing a home, and taking on a career and becoming a responsible member of a community. **Generativity vs. Stagnation**–Remain productive with career, family and community social participation, and adjust to physical changes of middle age. **Ego integrity vs. Despair**–Content that they have played a meaningful part in the lives of those around them, adjust to changes in physical strength and find satisfactory living arrangements.
   How has this health problem interfered with growth and development?

♦ 5. Health Care Providers
   What is the patient/family current level of understanding of the health problem?
   Are they satisfied with the care they are receiving?

♦ 6. Self-esteem and Body Image
   What changes in physical appearance?
   What changes in activity?

♦ 7. Cultural Experiences
   Religious preference and practices?
   Favorite foods?
   Years lived in the region?
   Travel outside of the region?

♦ 8. Gender: What were the gender speech behaviors of the patient?

*What communication techniques did you use with this patient?*_____

➤ *Note: It is not appropriate to ask the patient direct questions as you would during a history. Information is obtained by observing verbal and nonverbal behaviors and making inferences as you and the patient work toward accomplishing objectives.*

● Figure 6.3   Psychological- and sociocultural-assessment tool.

1. Current Emotional State

Assessment of a patient's emotional state must be continuous. You should be consciously aware of the patient's mood by monitoring her verbal and nonverbal behaviors. Is the patient feeling anxious, fearful, sad, hopeless, lonely, or out of control? These are very common emotional reactions. Emotions affect a person's ability to concentrate and can interrupt critical thinking abilities. Without the ability to concentrate, it is very difficult for the patient or family to analyze problems carefully or to learn about self-care during a patient education session. Emotions impair the individual's overall ability to communicate effectively. Nursing diagnoses that may apply include *Anxiety, Fear, Chronic Sorrow, Hopelessness, Grieving, Powerlessness,* and *Ineffective Coping.*

One of the most important patient-safe communication strategies you need to learn and use is empathy.[2] Empathy involves making it clear to the patient that you have recognized the emotion the patient expresses. You must interpret the patient's emotional response correctly and then verbally communicate that understanding to the patient. It is important to acknowledge and accept emotions. For example, you can simply say, "You seem sad." The purpose of empathy is to encourage ventilation by the patient, as well as for you to demonstrate acceptance of the patient's emotions.

2. Life Experiences

Use patient-safe communication strategies to assess and talk about changes in the patient's social roles as a result of health alterations.[2] The role alterations may be temporary or permanent, but the change will cause concern for patients and significant others. Talk with your patient about the circumstances surrounding how he came to be in the health-care setting and his perception of his current situation. For example, with a hospitalized patient, determine how his or her life has changed as a result of hospitalization; find out who is at home and how everyone in the family is managing while this family member is hospitalized. Consider how the problem has interfered with the patient's lifestyle and the goals the patient was trying to accomplish at the time the problem occurred. Also consider the type of work the patient does and the type of leisure activities he enjoys. Nursing diagnoses that may apply include *Interrupted Family Processes, Compromised Family Coping,* and *Ineffective Role Performance.*

3. Family and Significant Others

Social support is crucial to successful recovery. Take time to assess the ability of the patient's significant others to cope with the situation and to provide support for the patient. Family and friends commonly feel stress and strain when dealing with the patient's health problem and with the logistics of maintaining their home life and responsibilities. Nursing diagnoses that may apply include *Compromised Family Coping* and *Caregiver Role Strain.*

4. Growth and Development

Assess growth and development tasks as appropriate to the patient's age. The stages of growth and development were described by Erik Erikson[3] and included in Chapter 2. Consider how the patient's health problem is interfering with his ability to perform the appropriate growth and development tasks. For example, in young adulthood, tasks involve establishing intimacy and sexual roles, maintaining friendships, growing independent of parents, and establishing a career. A lengthy illness can severely disrupt all of these tasks. Nursing diagnoses that may apply include *Frail Elderly Syndrome* and *Risk for Delayed Development*

5. Relations With Health-Care Providers

The nature of a patient's relationship with health-care providers is very important to assess. It is important to know whether the health-care providers and the patient have been able to establish a working relationship and to develop mutual goals. The first consideration is the patient's ability to communicate. Some patients with impaired cognitive functioning—such as those with Alzheimer's disease—probably will not be able to communicate effectively and make rational decisions. Nursing diagnoses that may apply include *Impaired Verbal Communication, Impaired Memory,* and *Chronic Confusion.*

Thus, the family will be working closely with the health-care providers to discuss goals and outcomes.

Determine whether the patient and family understand the treatment regimen and whether they agree with and support it. Assess whether the patient and family have doubts or concerns about the plan. While providing care, look for evidence of clear or unclear communication between health-care providers and the patient or family. Stay alert to the level of understanding the patient and family have about the plan of care. You may want to ask the patient or a family member a general question, such as, "What has the doctor been saying to you about your diabetes?" or, "What have the nurses been teaching you about your diabetes?" After listening to the patient's answer, you could then follow with a general probing question, such as, "What do you think of all this?" Another good question to use to determine the patient's level of understanding for inpatient settings is, "Do you know when you are going home?" By staying alert and asking prudent questions, you can get a reasonable idea of the patient's and family's understanding of and feelings about the patient's problem. Nursing diagnoses that may apply include *Deficient Knowledge* and *Noncompliance.*

Patients often verbalize difficulty following the prescribed regimens and may fail to do them or fail to take action to reduce risk factors. The patient is unable to regulate and integrate a therapeutic regimen for the treatment of an illness and take actions to prevent additional complications. The goals and outcomes between the health-care provider and patient or family may not be mutual. For example, a patient with a lung condition may refuse to stop smoking. Not all patients are going to want to integrate all recommendations of health-care providers; they are diagnosed with *Ineffective Health Management.*[4] First, you must determine if the patient understands what is wrong and has been given explanations about how to stop smoking. You must also determine if the patient has the means to implement a smoking cessation plan if he decides he wants to do so. Ultimately, it is the patient's decision to agree or not to agree with any aspect of a therapeutic regimen.

Finally, another common relational problem involves turmoil over deciding what to do. The patient and family may have several health-care options from which they need to choose. For example, should a grandmother go to a nursing home, or should she move in with one of her children? Should the patient undergo chemotherapy for cancer? Health-care providers commonly guide patients in solving problems, especially as they examine their options. But it is the patient's and family's right to select the option that best suits them. Nursing diagnoses that may apply include *Decisional Conflict* and *Moral Distress.*

6. Self-Esteem and Body Image

It is important to assess the patient's self-concept pertaining to self-esteem and body image. Self-esteem is the value that people place on themselves. Because it is not appropriate to ask, "How is your self-esteem today?" you will need to infer it from the patient's body language, tone of voice, and words. As you interact with a patient, you can get clues to a person's sense of self-esteem by paying attention to expressions of feeling worthwhile or useless. People with high self-esteem usually can openly and honestly express what they think and feel. Even though patients have health problems, those with high self-esteem typically believe they are likable, capable of handling the challenge of the health problem, and effective in dealing with problems. According to Satir,[5] patients with low self-esteem placate, blame, compute, or distract. The placater tries to do whatever someone else says, not because she really wants to, but because she wants the other person to like her and not be mad at her. The blamer reacts to problems by yelling and giving orders. Beneath this exterior the person believes nobody loves or cares for her. The computer believes that showing emotions is a sign of weakness; this person lives by logic and rationalizations, although he feels very vulnerable. The distracter uses disruptions to get attention, has difficulty focusing on the issues at hand, and believes that no one cares about him. For a discussion of perception, self-concept, and self-esteem, with guidelines for effective patient-safe communication strategies, see Chapters 3 and 4 of Schuster and Nykolyn.[2]

Closely linked to self-esteem is body image. Body image refers to a person's feelings and attitudes towards the physical body. If he feels good about how he looks, it improves his self-esteem. If he feels bad about how he looks, it worsens his self-esteem. Many illnesses and the aging process alter the structure and functioning of the physical body, and body image disturbances result. Scars, deformities, amputations, weight gain or loss, and hair loss are examples of alterations that may lead to *Disturbed Body Image.* Body image disturbances may cause patients to be confused about how they perceive themselves. It takes time to integrate and accommodate changes in physical structure and function. Other nursing diagnoses that may apply include *Sexual Dysfunction, Ineffective Sexuality Pattern, Disturbed Personal Identity,* and *Chronic Low Self-Esteem.*

7. Cultural Experiences

It is important to assess the patient's cultural beliefs and practices. Cultural issues affect the plan of care. Many people are of mixed cultures. Everyone has beliefs and behaviors that have been passed down, although the origins of the beliefs and behaviors may not be known. Purnell and Paulanka's[6] model will be used as a guide for assessment of cultural experiences.

Purnell and Paulanka's model for cultural competence is an excellent tool for cultural assessment. The components of this model that are most relevant to cultural assessments of patients and their families, outlined in Box 6.1, are heritage, communication, family roles and organization, biocultural ecology, high-risk behaviors, nutrition, pregnancy and childbearing, death rituals, spirituality, health-seeking beliefs and behaviors, the culture of health-care practitioners, and cultural workforce issues.

Heritage

A person's country of origin commonly plays an important role in the development of her ideas and beliefs. For everyone except Native Americans, it is especially important to consider why the person, family, or cultural group migrated to North America. Most immigrate in hopes of a better life, but it may help you to know a more specific motivating factor. For example, migration may have resulted from political oppression, religious persecution, lack of job opportunities, or a natural disaster. Past economic and political experiences directly affect the individual's ideologies. It is important to consider the patient's and family's degree of orientation to their new culture and their familiarity with the health-care system and health-care providers.

Communication

In addition to the influence of language barriers on communication, also consider whether the patient feels comfortable sharing his thoughts and feelings. Cultural communication involves the amount of touch that is acceptable, personal space expected, eye contact deemed appropriate and the types and meanings of facial expressions used and body language displayed. Temporal relationships are also important to understand, because the expectations regarding punctuality vary among cultures. In addition, there are differing expectations regarding how to properly address people to maintain respect.

Family Roles and Organization

It is important to determine the dominant member of the household: the person in the family who is the spokesperson and decision-maker. In addition, the nature of the patient's nuclear family, extended family, and living space are important considerations in the plan of care, particularly with

Box 6.1	COMPONENTS OF PURNELL AND PAULANKA'S MODEL FOR ASSESSMENT OF CULTURE

- Heritage
- Communication
- Family roles and organization
- Biocultural ecology
- High-risk behaviors
- Nutrition
- Pregnancy and childbearing practices
- Death rituals
- Spirituality
- Health-seeking beliefs and behaviors
- Culture of health-care practitioners
- Cultural workforce issues

respect to the level of support the family gives to the member who needs health care. If family members cannot cope with the problem, other arrangements will need to be made.

Biocultural Ecology

Cultural groups have specific genetic, physical, and biologic characteristics, such as skin color, bone structure, and metabolism. These characteristics are noted in the general physical screening examinations. Health-care providers need to screen for specific health problems in different cultural groups because some diseases are genetically and environmentally transmitted. For example, sickle cell disease and diabetes occur with increased prevalence in particular ethnic groups. This information is routinely available on patient records and is part of the basic history screening examination.

High-Risk Behaviors

High-risk behaviors include the use of tobacco, alcohol, and recreational drugs; participation in high-risk physical activities; and lack of adherence to important health safety practices. Behaviors may vary with the cultural group and must be explored with each patient. Assessment of high-risk behaviors is typically part of the general screening health history.

Nutrition

A patient's diet is integral to many health problems and must be a topic of assessment. It is important that you become aware of the basic ingredients of native food dishes and preparation practices to provide culturally competent dietary counseling. Each cultural group has food preferences. The goal of dietary counseling is to select healthy foods from within the culturally preferred choices. Cultural meaning may be attached to foods that the patient eats or avoids. Food is often associated with cultural rituals.

Pregnancy and Childbearing Practices

Patients' beliefs and practices regarding fertility, birth control, pregnancy, birthing, and postpartum care vary widely and are based in part upon cultural background. For example, the selection of birth control methods, the roles of men in childbirth, the positions for delivering a baby, and preferred types of health practitioners (male or female, midwife or obstetrician) commonly differ among people of different cultural groups.

Death Rituals

It is important to identify culturally specific death rituals and mourning practices. Each culture has its own view of death, dying, and the afterlife. One of the goals of nursing a dying patient is to provide the means for a peaceful death. That can be accomplished only if you know the person's and family's death rituals. For example, a Catholic patient may want a priest to administer last rites, and a Muslim patient may want the bed positioned to face Mecca.

Spirituality

It is important to assess the dominant religion of an ethnic group, and to be aware of the patient's and family's use of activities such as prayer or meditation as a source of comfort. You should know how to contact the patient's religious leaders if the patient or family so desires. Keep in mind that spirituality does not always involve a specific religion: it involves beliefs about the meaning and purposes of life. The patient's and family's spirituality may be a source of emotional strength and sustenance through trying health-care situations.

Health-Seeking Beliefs and Behaviors

It is important to assess the predominant beliefs influencing a patient's health-care practices. Practices involve care of the sick, health promotion, and prevention. Cultures vary in their beliefs about pain, mental and physical handicaps, and chronic illness. Determine who will assume responsibility for care of the sick, and the role of health insurance in the culture. Included in this category are folklore practices that influence health behaviors. For example, blood transfusions or implantation of electrical devices may not be acceptable to a cultural group, although these are common medical practices.

Culture of the Health-Care Practitioners

When the health professional and patient are from different cultures, there may be a lack of trust if either person considers the other to be an outsider. The gender and the age of the health-care provider are also important to consider in providing culturally competent care. The status given to health-care providers and to the advice they give varies among cultures.

Cultural Workforce Issues

As a nurse, you will almost certainly work in a multicultural environment. Both patients and health-care providers come from a variety of cultural backgrounds. The primary factors related to work include language barriers, degree of assimilation, and autonomy issues. For example, difficulties may arise in the workplace from differing values placed on timeliness and punctuality, learning styles, personality styles, and levels of assertiveness. As you develop concept care maps for patients and families, cultural competence is needed not only with patients and their families but also with other health-care providers from different cultural backgrounds.

It is impossible to know the beliefs and practices of every culture, but health-care providers intent on providing culturally competent care continue to learn through traveling, reading, and attending events held by local ethnic and cultural organizations, as well as drawing on the expertise of colleagues. Health-care providers need to learn to conduct a cultural assessment effectively and then analyze and solve health-care problems of patients and their family members from the perspective of the patient's cultural group. Culturally competent health-care professionals are highly proficient in patient-safe communication.

It is particularly important that health-care providers refrain from making judgments about cultural behaviors and practices that they deem strange or "wrong." There are many ways to attain a mutual goal; to be philosophical, there are many paths to the same destination. Health-care providers must be resourceful and creative, and should tailor therapeutic regimens to suit the patient's culture. They must respect differences and appreciate the inherent worth of diverse cultures. The first step in becoming culturally competent is to become aware of your own values, attitudes, and beliefs. The learning activities at the end of this chapter are designed to put you in touch with your own ethnic background. There are numerous nursing diagnoses that may apply to culture, such as *Impaired Social Interaction*, *Spiritual Distress*, *Impaired Religiosity*, *Impaired Verbal Communication*, and *Risk-Prone Health Behavior*.

8. Gender

Gender differences in communication are partially derived from cultural background. Tannen's[7] work on gender differences in communication may help you to assess and respond appropriately to differing styles of speech in male and female patients. Communication patterns are culturally ingrained, although there may also be a biological basis for gender differences in communication. Tannen's research suggests that women speak, at least in part, to promote intimacy and to form communal connections, whereas men in their speech are more likely to focus on hierarchy, status attainment, and demonstration of status. As a nurse, you must learn to respond to patients based on the speech patterns you discern. General characteristics of male and female speech patterns are listed in Table 6.1. You may need to alter your communication patterns to suit the gender of your patient or teach your patient about gender differences in communication. A nursing diagnosis that may apply is *Readiness for Enhanced Communication*. For a more detailed discussion of how culture and gender issues are related to patient-safe communication strategies, see Chapter 5 in Schuster and Nykolyn's book Communication for Nurses: How to Prevent Harmful Events and Promote Patient Safety.[2]

Table 6.1 Traditional Gender Differences In Communication

Female	Male
Rapport talk	Report talk
Less adversarial	More adversarial
Cooperative overlapper	Talks alone
Listener	Information provider
Personal storytelling	Storytelling of human contests
Uses tag questions	Does not use tag questions
Conversational rituals: "I'm sorry" "Thanks"	Conversational rituals: Joking Teasing Sarcasm

The psychosocial and cultural assessment tool is to be used as a guide for collecting data and deriving appropriate nursing diagnoses. Bring this guide to clinical to assist you in the development of the psychosocial and cultural components of the concept care map. The guide entails eight basic categories of characteristics to assess as you work with the patient and family. Be aware, however, that more in-depth assessment of a particular area may be needed, depending on the situation. A vast amount of literature exists on each of the components of the psychosocial and cultural assessment. The guide barely scratches the surface of available knowledge, but it does provide a starting point for collecting psychosocial and cultural data.

Developing and Integrating the Psychosocial and Cultural Aspects of the Concept Care Map

Throughout the clinical day, you will assess, diagnose, plan, implement, and evaluate psychosocial and cultural problems. In this section, we will develop a clinical case study in detail to illustrate how you can integrate psychosocial and cultural data into your plan of care. A patient with breast cancer and a mastectomy will be used to illustrate this process.

Start with the initial patient profile database for the mastectomy patient who was presented in Chapter 3. The patient profile data base is reproduced for you in Figure 6.4. A student nurse collected this information on the day of surgery in preparation for care of the patient on the first postoperative day. A basic "sloppy copy" concept care map for steps 1 through 3 could look like what appears in Figure 6.5. Remember that concept care maps may vary in appearance; all the essential data from the profile in Figure 6.4 are on this sloppy copy in Figure 6.5.

This sloppy copy care map would need to be updated on arrival to the unit with the latest information on the patient, as described in Chapter 5. As you can see, the map includes data regarding physical pathology and physical assessment, medications, treatments, and laboratory results. Psychosocial and cultural problems are present, but not known in detail. The student

nurse could infer that the patient may have some form of depression because she is taking the drug Zoloft (sertraline) and because the removal of a breast is disfiguring and may influence her most intimate relationships. Therefore, there is some evidence to indicate the nursing diagnoses of *Disturbed Body Image* and *Chronic Sorrow* may be appropriate for this patient. There is little assessment data to support these diagnoses, so the nurse must continue the assessment during the clinical day. As the nurse continues to interact with the patient, she is able to do a more thorough continuation of the psychosocial and cultural assessment and gain more information regarding the cultural and developmental factors that will necessitate modification of the diagnoses and treatment strategies on the concept care map.

After the concept care map has been updated as described in Chapter 5, the student nurse will begin the initial key-assessments by checking the patient's vital signs, pain level, and dressing. *Acute Confusion* is a critical safety concern that is a priority assessment. Imagine that as the student nurse goes into the patient's room and says hello, the patient is confused and asks, "Where am I? Where is my son?" She begins to cry and says, "I want to go home." The student nurse may infer that the patient is probably anxious and sad because she is confused and tearful about where she is and who the nurse is. The student may infer that the patient may also feel very lonely and out of control. The student introduces herself, tells the patient where she is, takes the patient's hand, gives the patient some tissues, and explains quietly and calmly that she needs to check the blood pressure and dressing, and that she is going to take care of her. The student asks if the patient is hurting anywhere, and the patient responds, "No, I want my son Bobby." The student nurse tells the patient that she will try to find Bobby, and then she explains that she needs to check with the staff nurse and her faculty and that she will return very soon.

After leaving the room, the student nurse's initial impressions were as follows: this patient is anxious; she wants to go home, she is crying, and she misses her son. She also has acute confusion and is oriented only to her name. The student nurse adds these impressions to the concept care map, as shown in Figure 6.6. Confusion was originally included under the diagnosis of

Student Name: **MAB**

1) Date of Care: **12/24**	2) Patient Initials: **AL**	3) Age: **78** (face sheet)	3) Growth and Development **Ego integrity vs. Despair**	4) Gender: **F** (face sheet)	5) Admission Date: (face sheet) **12/3**

6) Reason for hospitalization (face sheet): Describe reason for hospitalization: (expand on back of page) *Medical Dx:* **Breast Cancer** *Pathophysiology:* *All signs and symptoms: Highlight those your patient exhibits*	7) Chronic illnesses (physician's history and physical notes in chart; nursing intake assessment and Kardex) **NIDDM** **Hypertension** **MI 1994**
8) Surgical procedures (consent forms and Kardex): Describe surgical procedure (expand on back of page) Name of surgical procedure: **Mastectomy** *Describe surgery:* **Right modified radical mastectomy**	

9) ADVANCE DIRECTIVES (NURSE'S ADMISSION ASSESSMENTS):

Living will: ☐ Yes ☐ No	Power of attorney: ☐ Yes ☐ No	Do not resuscitate (DNR) order (Kardex): ☐ Yes ☐ No

10) LABORATORY DATA:

Test	Normal Values	Admission 12/3	Date/Time 12/4	Date/Time	Reason for Abnormal Values
White blood cells (WBCs)		5.6	4.8		
Red blood cells (RBCs)					
Hemoglobin (Hgb)		11.2	11		
Hematocrit (Hct)		33.2	33.1		
Platelets		259,000			
Prothrombin time (PT)					
International normalized ratio (INR)					
Activated partial thromboplastin time (Aptt)					
Sodium Na					
Potassium K		2.8	2.8		
Chloride Cl					
Glucose (FBS/BS)		230	235		
Hemoglobin A1C					
Cholesterol					
Blood Urea Nitrogen (BUN)					
Creatinine					
Urine analysis (UA)					
Pre-albumin					
Albumin					
Calcium Ca					
Phosphate					
Bilirubin					
Alkaline phosphatase					
SGOT-Serum glutamic-oxyloacetic transaminase					
AST-Serum glutamic pyruvic transaminase					
CK					
CK MB					
Troponin					
B-natriuretic peptide BNP					
pH					
pCO_2					
pO_2					
HCO_3					

11) DIAGNOSTIC TESTS

Chest x-ray:	EKG:	Other abnormal reports:
Sputum or Blood Culture:	Other:	Other:

● Figure 6.4   Patient profile database: a surgical patient with mastectomy.

12) MEDICATIONS

List medications and times of administration (medication administration record and check the drawer in the carts for spelling). Include over-the- counter (OTC) products/herbal medicines.

Times Due	1000	0800	1000	1000
Brand Name		Lasix	Tenormin	Zoloft
Generic Name	heparin	furosemide	atenolol	sertraline
Dose	5000U	40mg	25mg	25mg
Administration Route	sq	po	po	po
Classification				
Action				
Reason This Patient is Receiving				
Pharmacokinetics	O P D 1/2 M E	O P D 1/2 M E	O P D 1/2 M E	O P D 1/2 M E
Contraindications				
Major Adverse Side Effects				
Nursing Implications				
Pt/Family Teaching				

Developed by P. Testa, YSU

Times Due	1000	1000	1000	q4h pm
Brand Name	Lanoxin	Ecotrin	K-dur	Tylenol
Generic Name	digoxin	aspirin	KCl	acetaminophen
Dose	01.25mg	1 tablet	20mg	650mg
Administration Route	po	po	po	po
Classification				
Action				
Reason This Patient is Receiving				
Pharmacokinetics	O P D 1/2 M E	O P D 1/2 M E	O P D 1/2 M E	O P D 1/2 M E
Contraindications				
Major Adverse Side Effects				
Nursing Implications				
Pt/Family Teaching				

Developed by P. Testa, YSU

ALLERGIES/PAINS

13) Allergies: **NKA** Type of Reaction: (medication administration record):	14) When was the last time pain medication given? (medication administration record) **Tylenol 6am (getting it sporadically)**
14) Where is the pain? **surgical incision** (nurse's notes)	14) How much pain is the patient in on a scale from 0-10? (nurse's notes, flow sheet): **5, confusion makes it unreliable**

TREATMENTS

15) List Treatments (Kardex): Rationale for treatments:
Dressing changes—sterile gauze & surgical bra, change qam
Ice to incision
Ted hose
IS q2h while awake
C&DB q2h while awake
I and O, & record q1h x 2

● Figure 6.4 Continued

16) Support services (Kardex) What do support services provide for the patient?
17) What does the consultant do for the patient?:

18) DIET/FLUIDS

Type of Diet (Kardex): **1800 ADA**	Restrictions (Kardex):	Gag reflex intact: ☐ Yes ☐ No	Appetite: ☐ Good ☐ Fair ☒ Poor	Breakfast **Eating** **Jello and tea only**	Lunch _____ %	Dinner _____ %
What type of diet is this?:						
What types of foods are included in this diet and what foods should be avoided?:						

Circle Those Problems That Apply:	
Prior 24 hours Fluid intake: (Oral & IV) **2100** Fluid output **1700** (flow sheet)	• Problems: swallowing, chewing, dentures (nurse's notes) • Needs assistance with feeding (nurse's notes) • Nausea or vomiting (nurse's notes) • Overhydrated or dehydrated (evaluate total intake and output
Tube feedings: Type and rate (Kardex)	on flow sheet • Belching: _____ • Other: _____ **Dentures and Needs Assistance Eating**

19) INTRAVENOUS FLUIDS (IV therapy record)

Type and Rate: **LR with 20 KCl 100/h**	IV dressing dry, no edema, redness of site: ☒ Yes ☐ No	Other:

20) ELIMINATION (flow sheet)

Last bowel movement: **None since surgery**	Foley/condom catheter: ☐ Yes ☒ No
Circle Those Problems That Apply:	

• Bowel: constipation, diarrhea, flatus, incontinence, belching
• Urinary: hesitancy, frequency, burning, incontinence, odor
• Other: _____
• What is causing the problem in elimination? _____

21) ACTIVITY (Kardex, flow sheet)

Ability to walk (gait):	Type of activity orders: **up as tolerated**	Use of assistance devices: cane, walker, crutches, prosthesis:	Falls-risk assessment rating: **7 high**
No. of side rails required (flow sheet) **4**	Restraints (flow sheet): ☒ Yes ☐ No **vest, wrist**	Weakness ☒ Yes ☐ No	Trouble sleeping (nurse's notes): ☒ Yes ☐ No

What does activity order mean?: _____ Why isn't the patient up ad lib?: _____ Would the problem cause weakness?: _____

PHYSICAL ASSESSMENT DATA

22) BP (flow sheet): **137/72** **152/100**	2) TPR (flow sheet): **97-52-20** **97.8-80-20**	23) Height: **5'5"** Weight: **190#** (nursing intake assessments)

24) NEUROLOGICAL/MENTAL STATUS:

LOC: alert and oriented to person, place, time (A&O x 3) confused, etc. **Alert & oriented to person only, became confused evening after surgery**	Speech: clear, appropriate/inappropriate **inappropriate**
Pupils: PERRLA	Sensory deficits for vision/hearing/taste/ smell **glasses**

● Figure 6.4   Continued

25) MUSCULOSKELETAL STATUS:

Bones, joints, muscles (fractures, contractures, arthritis, spinal curvatures, etc):	Extremity (temperature, edema (pitting vs. nonpitting) & sensation)
Motor: ROM x 4 extremities	
Ted hose/plexi pulses/compression devices: type:	Casts, splint, collar, brace:

26) CARDIOVASCULAR SYSTEM:

Pulses (radial, pedal) (to touch or with Doppler):	Capillary refill (<3s): ☐ Yes ☐ No	
Neck vein (distention):	Sounds: S1, S2, regular, irregular: Apical rate: **80**	Any chest pain:

27) RESPIRATORY SYSTEM:

Depth, rate, rhythm: **20**	Use of accessory muscles:	Cyanosis:	Sputum color, amount:	Cough: productive nonproductive	Breath sounds: clear, rales, wheezes **Clear, decreased in bases**
Use of oxygen: nasal cannula, mask, trach collar:	Flow rate of oxygen:	Oxygen humidification: ☐ Yes ☐ No	Pulse oximeter: _____ % oxygen saturation		Smoking: ☐ Yes ☐ No

28) GASTROINTESTINAL SYSTEM

Abdominal pain, tenderness, guarding; distention, soft, firm: **Soft & nondistended**	Bowel sounds x 4 quadrants: **Active 4 quads**	NG tube: describe drainage
Ostomy: describe stoma site and stools:	Other:	

29) SKIN AND WOUNDS:

Color, turgor: **Pink, poor turgor**	Rash, bruises: **Dry and chapped**	Describe wounds (size, locations): **Red & edematous**	Edges approximated: ☒ Yes ☐ No	Type of wound drains: **JP #1 25 ml** **JP #2 100 ml**
Characteristics of drainage: **serosanguineous**	Dressings (clean, dry, intact): **Clean, dry, intact**	Sutures, staples, steri-strips, other:	Risk for pressure ulcer assessment rating:	Other:

30) EYES, EARS, NOSE, THROAT (EENT):

Eyes: redness, drainage, edema, ptosis	Ears: drainage	Nose: redness, drainage, edema	Throat: sore
Psychosocial and Cultural Assessment			
31) Religious preference (face sheet) **Catholic**	32) Marital status (face sheet) **Widowed**	33) Health care benefits and insurance (face sheet): **Medicare**	
34) Occupation (face sheet) **Housewife**	35) Emotional state (nurse's notes) **Anxious, wants to go home, very talkative, does not respond to questions appropriately**		

● Figure 6.4   Continued

Risk for Injury, but as soon as the student talked to the patient, it was clearly evident that her confusion was a major patient care concern and needed special consideration.

The student nurse then discusses the situation with her faculty, who validates the diagnoses. Recognizing relationships between psychosocial and cultural diagnoses is very important. For example, as anxiety increases, confusion would also probably increase. It is important to recognize that physical problems affect and are interconnected with psychosocial and cultural problems, and vice versa. Humans respond in a holistic manner to health problems. Lines are drawn in Figure 6.6 show relationships among the patient's problems.

Key Problem #
Impaired Gas Exchange
-Breath sounds
decreased in bases
-Incentive spirometry

Key Problem #
Chronic Sorrow
Sertraline
(Zoloft)

Key Problem #
Disturbed Body Image
-Mastectomy

Key Problem #
Impaired Skin Integrity
-Wound: edematous,
red
2 drains: red drainage

Reason For Needing Health Care:
**Medical Diagnosis/Surgical Procedure:
Rt. modified radical mastectomy**

**Key Assessments: Pain, dressing,
drains, VS**

Key Problem #
Acute Pain
Acetaminophen (Tylenol)
Incision
5 on 10-point scale

Key Problem #
**Imbalanced Nutrition, Less
than Body Requirements**
-1800 ADA diet
-Poor appetite
-Needs help eating
-IV LR with KCl
-K-Dur
-Diabetic
-Blood glucose = 235
-5' 5", 190 lb
-Intake and
Output = 2100/1700
-Poor turgor

Key Problem #
**Decreased Cardiac
Output**
-Hx MI, hypertension
-137/72, 152/100
-Anemic
-H/H-11/32.1
-Aspirin (Ecotrin)
-Heparin
-Furosemide (Lasix)
-Potassium = 2.8
-K-Dur
-Valsartan (Diovan)

Key Problem #
**Risk for Injury, Impaired
Physical Mobility**
-Confusion
-Oriented to person only
-Inappropriate responses
to questions
-Pulled out IV and
restarted
-Restrained (vest/wrist)
-Wears glasses
-Falls risk: high

● Figure 6.5   Sloppy copy for a patient with a modified radical mastectomy; carry in pocket at
all times!

Before writing down outcomes and treatment strategies, you need to take note of how the student nurse intervened immediately when he recognized a problem in the above case study. What patient-safe communication strategies were used by the student nurse in the case study when the patient was crying and emotionally distraught above? An excellent discussion of patient-safe communication strategies with crying patients is included in Chapter 10 of Communication for Nurses: How to Prevent Harmful Events and Promote Patient Safety by Schuster and Nykolyn.[2]

Next, plan intervention strategies to help decrease *Anxiety* and *Acute Confusion*. The strategy list has been started for you, along with the goals and outcomes, in Figure 6.7. It is important to understand that psychosocial and cultural strategies are purposeful patient-safe communication strategies that are performed while continuing the assessment. As you read the continuation of the case study, identify the patient-safe communication strategies used by the student nurse as he continued the psychosocial and cultural assessment along with providing physical care.

The student nurse checks with the staff nurse, who says the patient's son Bobby just called in to check on her and is coming in soon. Bobby stated that his mother has not been

● Figure 6.6   Revised sloppy copy for the patient with a modified radical mastectomy (preconference), showing links between diagnoses.

confused at home, and that he cannot understand why this is happening now. The staff nurse assured Bobby that the doctors were trying to determine the cause of the confusion and that sometimes patients react in such a manner to anesthetics or medications. He also assured Bobby that his mother was being watched carefully. The staff nurse asked Bobby to bring in a family picture or some other object to help reorient his mother.

The student nurse goes back to the patient to finish his assessment and help the patient with breakfast. He makes small talk as he does the physical assessment, using distraction as the patient-safe communication strategy, talking about the patient's pretty blue robe that matches her blue eyes. The patient says that her daughter bought her the robe for her birthday. The patient's son comes in, and she brightens when she sees him and asks him to take her home.

Problem # ___ : Anxiety
General Goal: **Decreased Anxiety**

Predicted Behavioral Outcome Objective (s): The patient will...Talk about concerns, smile, rest peacefully... on the day of care.

Nursing Strategies	Patient Responses
1. Assess anxiety	1.
2. Use empathy	2.
3. Speak in quiet tone	3.
4. Active listening	4.
5. Caring touch	5.
6. Therapeutic humor	6.
7.	7.
8.	8.

Evaluation: Summarize patient progress toward outcome objectives:

_____

_____

Problem # _____ : Acute Confusion
General Goal: **Decreased Confusion**

Predicted Behavioral Outcome Objective (s): The patient will...not have injuries, and state why she is in the hospital... on the day of care.

Nursing Strategies	Patient Responses
1. Assess neurological status	1.
2. Reality orientation	2.
3. Orient time & place	3.
4. Use familiar objects	4.
5. Family member stays	5.
6. Use distraction-T.V.	6.
7. Give simple, single instructions	7.
8. Use consistency & repitition	8.

Evaluation: Summarize patient progress toward outcome objectives:

_____

_____

● Figure 6.7 Psychosocial and cultural nursing diagnoses, goals, objectives, strategies, and responses.

The student nurse continues the psychosocial and cultural assessment with the patient's son present and asks with whom she lives. Bobby explains that he and his son live with his mother, who cooks and cleans and takes care of them. He also explains that she is very active with the ladies' guild of St. Joseph's Catholic Church. He says that he wants to get her home as soon as possible. He brought in a school picture of his 15-year-old son and puts it on the night stand. The student nurse tells the patient what a handsome grandson she has, and the patient smiles.

The patient's son asks if the doctor has been in yet, because he wants to talk about why his mother was confused. The student nurse says he will go to page the doctor. When he returns to the room, he says the doctor will arrive shortly.

Based on these interactions, can you identify the important points of exchange between the student nurse and the patient's son that are components of the psychosocial and cultural assessment tool in Figure 6.3?

The student nurse next goes over the basic problems, and the goals, outcomes, and treatment strategies to correct the problems with both the patient and the patient's son. The patient and her son are active participants in the care planning process. As the student nurse goes over the plan, he can further assess cultural issues and modify the plan of care as needed. For example, the student may tell the patient and family that eating foods to promote wound healing is important. He asks what kinds of foods the patient likes to eat and finds out that the patient prefers the Italian food of her heritage as well as sweets of all kinds.

The student nurse discusses the need to keep the patient safe from falls and discusses her activity limitations and the use of restraints for safety. He also discusses the need to monitor vital signs and the care of the surgical wound. In addition, the student nurse discusses the need to improve oxygenation and to control pain.

The physician comes in and says that the patient may be reacting to the anesthetic and that her electrolytes are a little off and need to be corrected. The physician also says that the patient's wound is healing as anticipated. The son explains that he wants to take his mother home as soon as possible, and that he and his sister (who lives next door) would take care of her at home. He believes that once she gets back to her own home, his mother will not be as confused. The physician wants to keep the patient in the hospital for an additional day to regulate her electrolytes and to monitor her. The son agrees.

Recording Patient Responses

Patient responses to psychosocial and cultural issues should be recorded across from the nursing strategies in the same manner as that described in Chapter 5. Remember to record the patient's verbal and nonverbal behaviors in response to the strategies. For example, how does the patient respond to touch? Does she withdraw or smile? Also, write your impressions about the patient's progress toward or away from objectives. Did the patient's responses lead you to conclude that she was talking about her concerns? Was she able to state where she was and why she was there? Record the patient responses to the nursing strategies in the Patient Response column in Figure 6.7.

CHAPTER 6 SUMMARY

Psychosocial and cultural problems are often not known until you have face-to-face interactions with a patient. The focus of the initial concept care map is generally on physical information and treatments because, typically, only a small amount of psychosocial and cultural information is available in patient records. The bulk of information concerns physical pathology problems, medications, treatments, and laboratory results.

Assessment of a patient's psychosocial and cultural characteristics should be integrated throughout the time you work with the patient. Information collection is more informal than it is during a history and physical, and it should not be done through direct questioning and interviewing. It is accomplished by observing nonverbal behaviors, responses to touch, and facial mannerisms and having conversations with patients and family members.

There are eight major areas on which to focus when doing the psychosocial and cultural assessment, summarized in Box 6.2. The current emotional state assessment should be done continually and strategies performed as needed to promote emotional relaxation and comfort. Previous life experiences and how the problem disrupts the patient's lifestyle are important to consider, along with the effects of the problems on the family and significant others. Growth and development are disrupted by illness and interferes with a person's ability to accomplish expected tasks of growth and development. Self-esteem and body image can be altered when a health condition affects the patient's feelings of worth and feelings about their physical body. Cultural assessment involves the consideration of heritage, communication patterns, family roles and organization, biocultural ecology, high-risk behaviors, nutrition, pregnancy and childbearing practices, death rituals, spirituality, and health-seeking behaviors. Gender differences may result in differences in styles of speech.

Box 6.2   A SUMMARY OF GUIDELINES FOR PSYCHOSOCIAL AND CULTURAL ASSESSMENT

1. Current Emotional State

Use therapeutic communication to do an emotional assessment and find out the mood of the patient.

2. Life Experiences

Use therapeutic communication to talk with your patient about the circumstances surrounding the need for health care and about the patient's perception of the current situation. How has life changed as a result of the problem? How has this problem interfered with the life and the goals that the patient was trying to accomplish?

3. Family

How are family members coping with the situation? Are family members supportive? Who is performing the roles the patient cannot because of the health problem?

4. Growth and Development

What are the growth and developmental tasks relevant to the age of the patient? How has this health problem interfered with accomplishing those growth and developmental tasks?

5. Relations With Health-Care Providers

What have the doctor and other members of the health-care team been saying to the patient? When is the patient going home

(if applicable)? The aim is to determine the patient's current understanding of the problem. In addition, what type of relationship does the patient have with health-care providers? Are they able and willing to follow directions for treatments?

6. Self-Esteem and Body Image

As you talk with the patient, what inferences can be made regarding self-esteem and body image as a result of the health problems and the situation the patient is in? Does the patient appear to have confidence in her ability to care for herself, or does she have doubts and concerns? How accepting is she of the current situation?

7. Culture

As you talk with the patient, assess cultural beliefs and practices that are applicable to the current health-care situation. Key areas of assessment include responses to touch, personal space, eye contact, facial expressions, and body language. Determine who the dominant family members are and which family members have responsibility for health care. In addition, consider nutritional implications, spirituality, and cultural responses to pain.

8. Gender

What are the gender speech patterns present in the situation?

It is crucial for you to understand the relationship between psychosocial and cultural problems and physical problems. Psychosocial and cultural problems affect how physical problems are manifested and treated and vice versa. The concept care map serves to illustrate these relationships. You can demonstrate your knowledge of the integration of physical and psychosocial diagnoses by drawing lines to show relationships on concept care maps. The goals, outcomes, strategies, and responses involving psychosocial and cultural problems are written in the same format as described in previous chapters for physical problems.

Another important point to be made is that both physical and psychosocial and cultural assessments are ongoing throughout the clinical day. Changes in goals, outcomes, and strategies sometimes occur on a minute-to-minute basis because of new assessment information or a new evaluation of patient responses. The aim is to provide comprehensive holistic care.

LEARNING ACTIVITIES

1. In class, form groups of three or four and relate examples of patient-safe communication strategies you would use to develop a professional nurse-patient relationship. For example, empathy is a key patient-safe communication strategy used to develop a professional relationship with a patient and family. What would you say to show empathy? Other patient-safe communication strategies include emotionally supportive caring touch, therapeutic humor, active listening responses, responding with confirming messages, showing positive regard, perception checking, distraction, anticipatory guidance, reminiscence, and reality orientation, Assign the roles of nurse and patient to members of your group and role play each of these strategies. Discuss the nurse's strategies and the patient's specific verbal and nonverbal responses to the strategies.

2. To evaluate your own cultural background, do the mini–cultural assessment in Figure 6.8 at the end of this section. Get together in small groups to compare responses with classmates.

3. In class, form groups of three or four and relate clinical examples of psychosocial and cultural problems that you have encountered in your experiences as nursing students. Give an example to fit each of the categories of the guidelines for psychosocial, cultural, and developmental assessment. Give examples of alterations in emotional state, patient's life experiences, family, growth and development, relations with health-care providers, self-esteem, body image, culture, and gender. Elect a spokesperson to share examples with the entire class.

4. Practice developing psychosocial-cultural nursing diagnoses answering the following questions:

For each of these feelings, what is the psychosocial and cultural nursing diagnosis, and what are the verbal and nonverbal behaviors that indicate each emotion?

Anxious

Nursing diagnosis _____

Verbal _____

Nonverbals _____

Fearful

Nursing diagnosis _____

Verbal _____

Nonverbal _____

Sad

Nursing diagnosis _____

Verbal _____

Nonverbal _____

Hopeless

Nursing diagnosis _____

Verbal _____

Nonverbal _____

Lonely

Nursing diagnosis _____

Verbal _____

Nonverbal _____

Out of control

Nursing diagnosis _____

Verbal _____

Nonverbal _____

For each of the following roles, pretend the role has been disrupted due to a health problem. Write a possible psychosocial and cultural nursing diagnosis and a sentence about a situation in which this diagnosis would be appropriate. As a critical-thinking exercise, use a different diagnosis for each role alteration. There are a number of different diagnoses that could be appropriate, depending on the situation:

Worker

Nursing diagnosis _____

Rationale _____

Student

Nursing diagnosis _____

Rationale _____

Parent

Nursing diagnosis _____

Rationale _____

Husband/Wife

Nursing diagnosis _____

Rationale _____

Lover

Nursing diagnosis _____

Rationale _____

Friend

Nursing diagnosis _____

Rationale _____

Son/Daughter

Nursing diagnosis _____

Rationale _____

Sister/Brother

Nursing diagnosis _____

Rationale _____

Grandparent

Nursing diagnosis _____

Rationale _____

For each of the following psychosocial and cultural problems involving an interaction with the health-care provider, give a psychosocial and cultural nursing diagnosis. Write a sentence about why this diagnosis would be appropriate. As this is a critical-thinking exercise, use a different diagnosis for each situation.

The patient signs himself out of the hospital against medical advice.

Nursing diagnosis _____

Rationale _____

The family cannot decide whether or not to permit the patient to have a feeding tube.

Nursing diagnosis _____

Rationale _____

The family cannot handle all the care required for the ventilator-dependent child at home.

Nursing diagnosis _____

Rationale _____

The cardiac patient states that she has no time to do her exercise prescription.

Nursing diagnosis _____

Rationale _____

For each of the following situations, which involve changes in body image or self-esteem, give a possible psychosocial and cultural nursing diagnosis, and write a sentence about why this diagnosis would be appropriate. Use a different diagnosis for each alteration.

The patient refuses to look at the appendectomy scar.

Nursing diagnosis _____

Rationale _____

The patient with a heart attack states, "I'm just no good anymore. I'll never be able to go back to my old job."

Nursing diagnosis _____

Rationale _____

The patient admits, "I'm so ashamed of the way I look without my hair since the chemotherapy."

Nursing diagnosis _____

Rationale _____

The patient says, "I haven't been outside this apartment for 6 months because I'm a cripple and I don't want anyone to see me."

Nursing diagnosis _____

Rationale _____

For each of the following examples of cultural nursing care problems, give a possible psychosocial and cultural nursing diagnosis and write a sentence about why this diagnosis would be appropriate. Use a different diagnosis for each alteration.

The patient says she can't understand how God could have let this happen to her.

Nursing diagnosis _____

Rationale _____

An East Indian woman comes by ambulance into labor and delivery and screams with each contraction. She doesn't understand English, and there is no interpreter available. Her husband is on the way to the hospital.

Nursing diagnosis _____

Rationale _____

A Jehovah's Witness patient with a hemoglobin of 5 is actively bleeding and is refusing blood.

Nursing diagnosis _____

Rationale _____

5. Practice patient-safe communication strategies by completing the exercise below.

Following are gender communication examples. Specify whether each of the following is a typical male or female pattern of communication. Write why you think so and specify what you would say in reply.

The physician comes into the room, says hello, and asks, "What's going on with Mrs. G.?"

_____

The nurse says to the patient, "It's time to get up to sit in a chair, don't you think so?"

_____

The patient says to the nurse, "I'm sorry to be such a bother to you."

_____

Mini Cultural Assessment: Please assess yourself, then exchange views with others from similar and different cultural backgrounds.

1. What people from cultural/ethnic groups have you become friends with?
2. In what country were you born?
3. In what countries did your ancestors originate on your mother's and father's sides of your family?
4. How closely do you associate with your parents and grandparents?
5. Whom do you consider your family? Relatives, friends, pets?
6. How important is your family to you?
7. In your family, who takes care of infants and children? Who spends the most time taking care of them?
8. In your family, who takes care of the sick or elderly? Who spends the most time taking care of them?
9. Describe your thoughts and feelings about marriage.
10. Describe your thoughts and feelings about childbearing.
11. Should a mother nurse her baby in public or private? Should babies be breastfed?
12. The environment refers to the planet Earth and the communities in which people live. Should we preserve or use the resources? Should we recycle?
13. What is the meaning of life? Explain. Why are people put on Earth?
14. What do you think about death? What happens when you die?
15. How important is punctuality to you? Should people be on time?
16. What do you think about the past? Is what happened in the past relevant to the present?
17. What do you think about the present? Should we live "for the moment"?
18. What do you think about the future? What should the future bring?
19. Is money and having status important?
20. Who does the cooking, cleaning, yard work, care maintenance in your family?
21. How are decisions made in your family? Are steps of problem solving followed in your family? Explain how decisions are made in your family.
22. What place do elderly relatives have in your life?
23. Is the sex of a baby important? Are girls and boys treated differently as they grow?
24. What rules govern sexual activity for a man? For a woman?

● Figure 6.8   Mini-cultural assessment. (Adapted with permission from Schuster PM. *Communication: The Key to the Therapeutic Relationship.* Philadelphia, Pa: F.A. Davis; 2000.)

REFERENCES

1. The Joint Commission, 2004: Sentinel Event Statistics, June 29, 2004. Cited by: Leonard M, Graham S, Bonacum D. The human factor: The critical importance of effective teamwork and communication in providing safe care. *Quality and Safety in Health Care*. 2004;13:i85-i90.

2. Schuster PM, Nykolyn L. *Communication for Nurses: How to Prevent Harmful Events and Promote Patient Safety*. Philadelphia, Pa: F.A. Davis; 2010.

3. Erikson EH. *The Life Cycle Completed*. New York, NY: Norton; 1998.

4. NANDA International. *NANDA Nursing Diagnoses: Definitions and Classification, 10th ed. 2015–2017*. Herdman TH, ed. Chichester, United Kingdom: Wiley-Blackwell; 2014.

5. Satir V. *New Peoplemaking*. Mountain View, Calif: Science and Behavior Books; 1988. (Seminal Book)

6. Purnell LD, Paulanka BJ. *Transcultural Health Care: A Culturally Competent Approach*. 4th ed. Philadelphia, Pa: F.A. Davis; 2012.

7. Tannen D. *You Just Don't Understand: Women and Men in Conversation*. New York, NY: Quill; 2001.

7

CONCEPT CARE MAPS AS THE BASIS OF DOCUMENTATION AND PHONE CONVERSATIONS WITH PHYSICIANS

OBJECTIVES

1. List purposes of documentation.

2. Describe the relationships between the American Nurses Association standards of professional nursing practice, the American Nurses Association documentation standards, and concept care maps.

3. Specify the basic content of nursing care documentation.

4. Compare documentation formats for standardized forms and narrative progress notes.

5. Identify basic criteria that guide documentation.

6. Use the concept care map to identify content for documentation.

7. Describe the purpose of HIPAA documentation.

8. Use the concept care map to develop the SBAR to communicate with physicians and document the conversation.

The purposes of this chapter are to provide basic information about the process of basic documentation and to explain the use of concept care maps as guides for documentation. Documentation, also known as charting, is the legal record of written communication of all patient care activities from each health-care provider involved in the patient's care. It is crucial that nursing students know how to document accurately and efficiently. This chapter provides a very basic guide to documentation;

nursing students will be given very specific documentation guidelines during clinical rotations to differing health-care facilities and also as they change units within the same health-care facility.

Nurses are legally accountable for following nursing standards of care, and documentation is the written evidence that standards of care were followed. This is also the situation for all other health-care providers involved in patient care. All providers must follow standards of care for their own professional disciplines and provide written evidence that standards were met. Should there be a malpractice claim, patient records will be subpoenaed in court, and this legal record may be used as evidence of the health-care services provided and the patient's responses to those services.

Administrators of health-care agencies use patient records to conduct quality assurance audits to monitor the effectiveness and efficiency of all services. Written documentation is needed to ensure quality of patient care by supplying evidence to administrators that health-care providers are doing their jobs. Health-care administrators are interested in maintaining accreditation and enforce strict standards of documentation. Administrators are also focused on collection of money for services provided from insurance companies, managed care organizations, Medicare, and Medicaid for services provided. The amount of reimbursement is based on documentation. Failure to correctly document provided services results in lack of appropriate reimbursement.

Everything that was written on the concept care map is documented somewhere in the patient records. Information must be documented concerning all medical and nursing diagnoses that have been identified in the concept care map, through use flow sheets, progress notes, or care plans. Steps 1, 2, and 3 of concept care mapping, involving development of the diagram, will be used as the basis for documentation of assessment data. Step 4, involving outcomes and strategies, will be used to guide documentation of implementation of nursing strategies to attain outcomes. Step 5, notes on the evaluation of patient responses to nursing strategies, will be used to guide documentation of patient responses and progress toward outcome objectives. Documentation is a challenge for every

health-care provider. Formats for documentation and the exact procedures for documentation are in a constant state of flux. However, the concept care maps are very useful tools to help you focus on the basic content of what must be documented.

What to Document

The primary objective is to provide evidence that practice standards have been upheld. It is also a form of communication with other health-care providers and a way to ensure the best, most seamless health-care provision possible. Assessments, diagnoses, outcomes, strategies, and patient responses must be documented for each encounter with a patient.

Nurses must understand the relationships between documentation standards and care standards of the American Nurses Association (ANA)[1] and concept care maps. Linkages between standards of care, documentation standards, and concept map care plans as shown in Figure 7.1. Concept care maps facilitate documentation because they are cohesive, written, individualized summaries of patient care based on professional standards of practice.

In summary, documentation standards require patient care assessment data be documented in retrievable form. Nursing and medical diagnoses must be included and must be documented in a manner that facilitates the determination of expected patient outcomes. Patient outcomes need to be documented as measurable outcome objectives. There must be a written plan of care with specified strategies and active patient participation in development of the care plan. All strategies that are implemented and patient responses to the strategies must be documented. All reassessments and revisions in diagnoses, outcomes, and the plan of care are documented as well.

Where to Document

Everything on the care map needs to be documented somewhere. It is initially overwhelming to think that *everything* has to be recorded in medical records. However, not

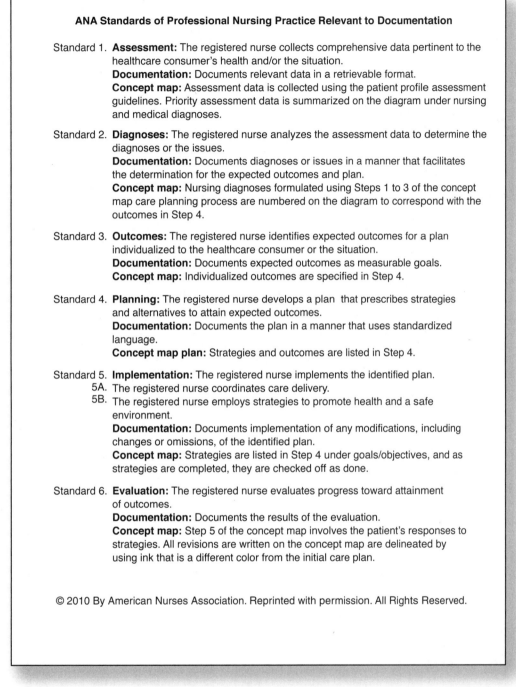

ANA Standards of Professional Nursing Practice Relevant to Documentation

Standard 1. **Assessment:** The registered nurse collects comprehensive data pertinent to the healthcare consumer's health and/or the situation.
Documentation: Documents relevant data in a retrievable format.
Concept map: Assessment data is collected using the patient profile assessment guidelines. Priority assessment data is summarized on the diagram under nursing and medical diagnoses.

Standard 2. **Diagnoses:** The registered nurse analyzes the assessment data to determine the diagnoses or the issues.
Documentation: Documents diagnoses or issues in a manner that facilitates the determination for the expected outcomes and plan.
Concept map: Nursing diagnoses formulated using Steps 1 to 3 of the concept map care planning process are numbered on the diagram to correspond with the outcomes in Step 4.

Standard 3. **Outcomes:** The registered nurse identifies expected outcomes for a plan individualized to the healthcare consumer or the situation.
Documentation: Documents expected outcomes as measurable goals.
Concept map: Individualized outcomes are specified in Step 4.

Standard 4. **Planning:** The registered nurse develops a plan that prescribes strategies and alternatives to attain expected outcomes.
Documentation: Documents the plan in a manner that uses standardized language.
Concept map plan: Strategies and outcomes are listed in Step 4.

Standard 5. **Implementation:** The registered nurse implements the identified plan.
5A. The registered nurse coordinates care delivery.
5B. The registered nurse employs strategies to promote health and a safe environment.
Documentation: Documents implementation of any modifications, including changes or omissions, of the identified plan.
Concept map: Strategies are listed in Step 4 under goals/objectives, and as strategies are completed, they are checked off as done.

Standard 6. **Evaluation:** The registered nurse evaluates progress toward attainment of outcomes.
Documentation: Documents the results of the evaluation.
Concept map: Step 5 of the concept map involves the patient's responses to strategies. All revisions are written on the concept map are delineated by using ink that is a different color from the initial care plan.

● Figure 7.1   ANA standards of professional nursing practice relevant to documentation. (©2010 By American Nurses Association. Reprinted with permission. All rights reserved.)

everything has to be personally typed into a computer or written down by your own hand, word by word. Health-care agencies provide nurses with standardized forms to accomplish the daunting task of documentation (Fig. 7.2). In addition, succinct written narrative comments are recorded on progress note forms (Fig. 7.3).

Forum
HEALTH

MEDICAL/SURGICAL FLOW SHEET   DATE _____

V S **I I** **T G** **A N** **L S**	**TIME**	
	Temperature	
	Pulse	
	Respirations	
	Blood Pressure	
A **S** **S** **E** **S** **S** **M** **E** **N** **T**	**MENTAL STATUS**	
	PAIN	
	RESP STATUS	Breath Sounds
		Type
	G.I. STATUS	Bowel Sounds
		Abdomen
	PERIPHERAL VASCULAR STATUS	Radial
		Dorsalis Pedis
	INTEGUMENTARY STATUS	Color/Temp
		Wound/Lesion
	DUP SCORE **Every Monday**	
	IV SITE_____ /RATE	
	IV SITE_____ /RATE	
	MOBILITY	
	FALLS SCORE **Every Monday**	
	R.N. INITIALS	
I **N** **T** **E** **R** **V** **E** **N** **T** **I** **O** **N** **S**	**ACTIVITY/SAFETY**	Bedrest
		Turn
		ROM
		Leg Exercises
		Chair
		Ambulation
		Bathroom
		BSC
		Bedpan/Urinal
		Siderails/Call Light
		HOB ↑
	HYGIENE	Bath/Shower
		HS/Back Care
		Mouth Care
		Cath Care
	DIET	Consumed
		Method
		NPO/HS Snack
	TUBE FEEDING	Rate
		Residual Check
		Tube Placement Check
	TREATMENTS	DB and Cough
		TED Hose/Binder
	RESTRAINT CHECK	Level_____

(Peripheral Vascular Status row marked with repeated R L columns)

● Figure 7.2   Sample flow sheet. (From Forum Health, Youngstown, Ohio, with permission.)

													TIME	
													Temperature	V S
													Pulse	I I
													Respirations	T G
													Blood Pressure	A N L S
													MENTAL STATUS	
													PAIN	
													Breath Sounds RESP STATUS	A
													Type	
													Bowel Sounds GI STATUS	S
													Abdomen	S
R	L	R	L	R	L	R	L	R	L	R	L		PERIPHERAL	E
													Radial VASCULAR STATUS	S
													Dorsalis Pedis	S
													Color/Temp INTEGUMENTARY	M
													Wound/Lesion STATUS	
													DUP SCORE Every Monday	E
													IV SITE_____/RATE	
													IV SITE_____/RATE	N
													MOBILITY	
													FALLS SCORE Every Monday	T
													R.N. INITIALS	
													Bedrest ACTIVITY/SAFETY	
													Turn	
													ROM	
													Leg Exercises	I
													Chair	N
													Ambulation	
													Bathroom	T
													BSC	
													Bedpan/Urinal	E
													Siderails/Call Light	R
													HOB ↑	V
													Bath/Shower HYGIENE	E
													HS/Back Care	
													Mouth Care	N
													Cath Care	
													Consumed DIET	T
													Method	
													NPO/HS Snack	I
													Rate TUBE FEEDING	O
													Residual Check	
													Tube Placement Check	N
													DB and Cough TREATMENTS	
													TED Hose/Binder	S
													RESTRAINT CHECK	

CODES

* Needs further explanation

Pulse
AP - Apical pulse
R - Regular
I - Irregular*

Temperature
AX - Axillary temp
R - Rectal temp
T - Tympanic

Mental Status
A = Alert/0x3
S = Sleeping
O = Other*

Pain
0 = None
Scale 1-10*

Bowel Sounds
N = Normal
0 = Absent*
↑ = Increased*
↓ = Decreased*

Pulses
0 = Absent*
1+ = Weak*
      Thready
2+ = Decreased*
3+ = Normal
4+ = Bounding

Mobility
N = Normal
I = Impaired*

Activity/Hygiene/Turn/Pos
L = Left Side
R = Right Side
B = Back
P = Prone

Consumed
G = Good 80-100%
F = Fair 60-80%
P = Poor 60%

Resp. Type
N = Normal
S = Shallow*
D = Deep
L = Labored

Breath Sounds
C = Clear
Rh= Rhonchi*
Ra= Rales*
Wz= Wheeze*

Abdomen
S = Soft
D = Distended*
F = Firm*

Skin Temp
W = Warm/Dry
C = Cool
D = Diaphoretic*

Skin Color
N = Normal
C = Cyanotic*
J = Jaundiced*
O = Other*

Wound/Lesion
N = None
O = Other*

Tube Feeding
C = Continuous
B = Bolus
I = Intermittent

S = Self
A = Assist
C = Complete

Method
S = Self
A = Assist
F = Feed

Level I Restraint Check includes:
• Visual observation
• Restraint placement
• *Other

Level II & III Restraint Check includes:
• Visual observation
• Restraint placement
• Color/Temperature Check
• Restraint Release for 10 min. q 2 h
• Activity/ROM
• The offer for toileting and norishment/fluids
• Mental Status
• *Other

Initials	Signature	Shift R.N.

7301005 Rev. 12/97

● Figure 7.2   Continued

Forum
H E A L T H

NURSES NOTES
USE "MIDNIGHT LINE" FOR DATING
THE NEW DAY

Addressograph

Date/Time

HOUR	P.R.N. and Stat Medication	NOTES
9-8-15		
0800		Reports pain in surgical incision area "5" on "10"
		point scale, requests pain medication. N Direnzo, YSU, SN_____
0810		Given 2 vicodin for pain w/ instruction on use
		of visual imagery exercises & slow deep breathing.
		N Direnzo, YSU, SN _____
0900		Reports pain is now "2". N Direnzo, YSU, SN _____

7301811

● Figure 7.3   Sample nurse's notes.

Standardized Paper or Computerized Forms

You must become familiar with the standardized forms or computerized forms that provide the basis of documentation in each health-care facility. Standardized forms increase consistency and the completeness of information gathered and decrease time spent in documentation. Typical formats of standardized forms include checklists and fill-ins with space for a few words. Blank sections are provided on standardized forms to expand on and clarify information to allow individualization of care. As you gain clinical experience at different health-care agencies, you will note many similarities in the contents of standardized forms. Although contents are similar, the layout varies. You will also be expected to record documentation information on the flow sheets and progress notes used by the health-care facility.

Documentation Standards for Assessment and Reassessment

There are many standardized forms for the assessment and reassessment of patients to help you meet documentation standard 1, that all data is documented in a retrievable form. There are standardized forms used for the continual assessment and evaluation of the care of patients, which include history and physical admission assessments and specialized, customized key assessments that occur on an ongoing basis. When assessments are ongoing, they are considered reassessments. You can also think of the reassessments as data for continued evaluation of patient responses to nursing strategies. The terminology gets a bit confusing, but after an initial assessment, nurses continue to assess in order to evaluate responses to nursing strategies.

As patients enter the inpatient or outpatient health-care system for the first time, there will be a comprehensive history and physical done on admission, with subsequent key reassessments customized to the health problems. For example, for a patient with hypertension, after the initial complete history and physical, the focus of key subsequent assessments will be on the cardiovascular system. Each area of care, such as medical units, surgical units, outpatient clinics, pediatric clinics, and geriatric units, will conduct a complete history and physical and then focus follow-up/evaluations by collecting data specific to the type of patient care services provided by the facility.

Assessments and Standardized Flow Sheets

Flow sheets are a special type of standardized form used for frequent assessments or reassessments. Nurses always start with a baseline assessment. Subsequent assessments of the same parameter are considered reassessments, but may also be considered evaluation data. For example, assessments of neurological checks and vital signs are tracked with flow sheets. Flow sheets have formats that allow key data to be seen either in columns or rows and tracked over time. Flow sheets allow easy comparisons to determine trends in assessment data over time. A sample flow sheet is shown in Figure 7.2.

Linking Concept Care Maps to Documentation of Assessment and Reassessments

The concept care map is useful to guide ongoing assessments, reassessments, and evaluations on agency standardized documentation forms. Step 5 of the concept care map contains information you have written on patient responses, which are reassessments of what was initially assessed using the patient profile database. Make sure you know where to document assessment and reassessment information on the agency's standardized forms.

Documentation Standards for Nursing Diagnoses and Care Plans

The purpose of developing care plans is to communicate diagnoses, goals, and outcomes of care; coordinate patient care; and ensure continuity of care. Many health-care agencies have developed standardized care plans for patients with specific diagnoses to decrease paperwork and to meet accreditation standards for practice and documentation.[2] Historically, health-care agencies and nursing schools developed an individualized care plan that had four columns that included nursing diagnoses; patient/family outcomes, nursing strategies, rationales for strategies, and evaluation of patient outcomes (see Fig. 7.4).

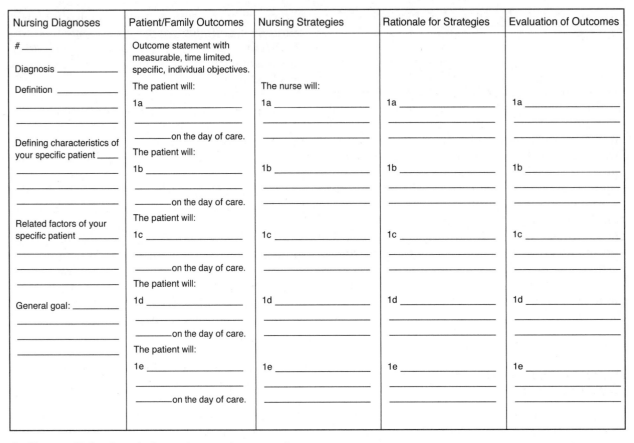

● Figure 7.4   Sample four-column patient care plan.

Through use of standardized care plans, nurses need only check, date, and sign appropriate columns in the plan, to save time writing about routine outcomes, strategies, rationales, and evaluation of outcomes. Space is usually provided on the standardized forms for individualized outcomes and strategies. A sample standardized care plan from a hospital is shown in Figure 7.5.

Standardized care plans are useful to nurses and student nurses who are inexperienced in caring for patients with particular diagnoses because expected outcomes and strategies are clearly evident. In each agency you are assigned for clinical experiences, you need to locate and study standardized care plans, which may be computerized or preprinted. If care plans are not available, there are numerous up-to-date standardized nursing care plan texts available as well as medical-surgical texts containing standardized plans of care to guide you in developing the individualized concept care maps. Experienced nurses

have the outcomes, strategies, and rationales ingrained from practice, and thus have little use for standardized plans of care. There are still numerous complaints from nurses that standardized nursing care plans are just extra paper work to check, date, and sign.

The current trend in care planning is for agencies to develop and use the standardized interdisciplinary care plans called *critical* or *clinical pathways*. These are based on outcomes for specific patient problems, such as a knee replacement. They have been developed by teams of health-care providers involved in the care of a specific patient population. As with other standardized care plans, nurses need only check, date, and sign the appropriate columns of the care plan.

Linking Concept Care Maps to Documentation on Standardized Column Care Plans
Concept care maps organize and individualize nursing care delivery and increase learning, and should

INITIATED

| Date: |
| Time: |
| RN: |

DISCONTINUED

| Date: |
| Time: |
| RN: |

INITIATED		NURSING DIAGNOSIS PATIENT CARE PROBLEM	PATIENT OUTCOMES	EVALUATED		NURSING INTERVENTIONS	RESOLVED	
Date	RN			Date	RN		Date	RN
		① Disturbed Body Image related to body image change and value in reproductive organ.	Pt will demonstrate adaptive responses related to body image: Pt will ask appropriate questions. State correct information related to procedures and prognosis. State she discussed concerns with partner. _____ Date			① Encourage pt's comments and questions about surgery, prognosis. ② Reinforce correct information and provide factual information. ③ Encourage verbalization with significant other. ④ Discuss hormone replacement therapy. ⑤ Implement pre-op protocol. ⑥ _____ ⑦ _____		
		② Pain related to surgical incision.	Verbalizes minimal discomfort or absence of pain. (ongoing) _____ Date Progress from IV/IM meds to PO pain meds by second post-op day. _____ Date			① Implement acute pain protocol. ② Teach pain rating scale to patient (1–10). ③ Reinforce splinting technique if abdominal incision present. ④ Assist pt in assuming a position of comfort. ⑤ Keep foley catheter free from pulling. ⑥ _____ ⑦ _____		

● Figure 7.5   Sample standardized care plan. (Modified from Forum Health, Youngstown, Ohio, with permission.)

be used in combination with standardized column care plans. At the clinical agency, use the concept care map to individualize the standardized care plans. If there are diagnoses on the diagram that are not included in standardized plans, add them to the standardized plan with appropriate outcomes and strategies.

Documentation Standards for Implementation of Nursing Strategies

Standard treatments, medications, and intravenous (IV) fluids are documented on flow sheets. Examples of standard treatments in hospital settings include bath, back care, and oral care. Space is provided on standardized forms for additional treatments to individualize the plan of care. Nursing strategies such as administering medications and IV fluids are very important nursing activities, and they must be documented carefully using medication and IV administration flow sheets. For example, an antibiotic administered over 3 days is tracked from time to time and day to day across a row of a medication flow sheet. All prn (as needed) medications will be documented on the flow sheets and also expanded upon in the narrative notes. Documentation of treatments, medications, and IV therapy is done by listing the dates and times in the appropriate spaces on the flow sheets.

Linking Concept Care Maps to Documentation on Flow Sheets

Strategies are listed on the front of the diagram under each diagnosis. In addition, strategies are listed in step 4 of the concept care map. All ongoing treatment strategies should be listed on the treatment flow sheet. Medications and IVs are highlighted on the front of the diagram and documented on flow sheets. Specific strategies to alleviate problems will be included with more detailed narrative documentation of specific problems. A sample flow sheet with assessments and strategies is shown in Figure 7.2.

Documentation of Specific Problems

Standardized forms for assessments, strategies, and reassessments or evaluations save a lot of time and organize information. There is not enough room on the forms to go into detail for problems. Details of specific problems, strategies, and patient responses are expanded upon using progress notes (also called *narrative notes*), shown in Figure 7.3.

The content of documentation of specific problems can be determined easily using the concept care map diagram of problems as a guide. Each nursing diagnosis must be described in the progress notes. For each nursing diagnosis, documentation can be done in three steps. First, describe the problem; second, write intervention strategies; and last, evaluate the patient's responses.[3]

Progress Note: Problem

First, list the nursing diagnosis and then describe the problem by writing down abnormal assessment data that support the diagnosis. Abnormal assessment data are located on the diagram of the concept care map under each diagnosis. In addition, assessment data is located in step 5, patient responses/evaluation of the concept care map. For example: .

> *2/11/15 8 a.m. problem: Pain (surgical incision)*
> *Reports pain in surgical incision area "5" on 10-point scale, requests medication. N. DiRenzo, YSU, SN*

Note that the date and the time are written first, followed by the diagnosis and assessment data. In this example, the assessment data is subjective, because it indicates what the patient reported about pain.

Progress Note: Intervention Strategies

Second, describe what was done to alleviate the problem. Write all strategies and instructions given to the patient. Strategies are listed under the diagnoses on the diagram of the concept care map. In addition, strategies are listed in step 4 of the concept care map.

> *8:10 a.m. Given 2 Vicodin (hydrocodone/ acetaminophen) for pain w/instruction on visual imagery exercises. N. DiRenzo, YSU, SN*

Progress Note: Evaluation

Third, describe the patient's response to the nursing strategies that were done. This entails reassessment and evaluation of the initial assessment data. Evaluation of patient responses to nursing strategies occurs in step 5 of the concept care map.

> *9:00 a.m.: Reports pain is now "2." N. DiRenzo, YSU, SN*

In the actual progress notes with explanations deleted, the entry would look like this:

> *2/11/15 8 a.m. problem: Pain (surgical incision)*
> *Reports pain around surgical incision "5" on 10-point scale, requests medication. N. DiRenzo, YSU, SN*
> *8:10 a.m.: Given 2 Vicodin (hydrocodone/acetaminophen) for pain w/instruction on visual imagery. N. DiRenzo, YSU, SN*
> *9:00 a.m.: Reports pain is now "2." N. DiRenzo, YSU, SN*

The preceding example shows the basics of documentation, but sometimes problems do not resolve quite as easily. In the next example, the initial strategies do not work to alleviate the problem, so more strategies are performed and patient responses are again evaluated (reassessed):

> *2/11/15 8 a.m. problem: Constipation (postoperative decreased GI motility)*
> *Reports unable to have BM in 3 days and abdominal discomfort is "3" on a 10-point scale, belching and passing flatus, bowel sounds present 4 quadrants. N. DiRenzo, YSU, SN*
> *8:10 a.m. Given 30 cc MOM (magnesium hydroxide), instructed to drink more water, and given warm tea to drink. N. DiRenzo, YSU, SN*
> *10 a.m. Bowel assessment unchanged from 8 a.m. N. DiRenzo, YSU, SN*

Unfortunately, constipation is not alleviated by using milk of magnesia or by drinking water and tea; additional strategies are therefore needed. It frequently occurs that you will need to continue to work on a problem throughout the day. The nurse has reassessed/evaluated the outcome, and now has to intervene and document additional strategies. There is an ongoing problem, so the evaluation becomes a reassessment and leads directly to the need for additional strategies. This is followed by reassessment/evaluation in the following example.

Write Another Progress Note: Additional Strategies

What was done next?
> *10:10 a.m. Given Fleet enema. N. DiRenzo, YSU, SN*

Write Another Progress Note: Evaluation

Patient response now?

> *10:15 a.m. Large brown formed BM per bedside commode. Patient reports feeling better, discomfort "0." N. DiRenzo, YSU, SN*

This documentation system of using standardized forms with progress notes to give details on problems has been termed *documentation by exception*; also termed a problem-oriented approach.[4] Checklists and fill-ins are useful to quickly record assessments, strategies, and evaluations. Problems identified are then expanded in the progress notes. There is no need to write details about assessments/evaluations that are within normal limits; it is only necessary to write about the exceptions to the norm. It is very important to be able to provide an in-depth description of the problems, with strategies and evaluation of patient responses to nursing strategies.

Mnemonics (memory aids) for writing progress notes include DAR and SOAPIER. The information contained in the entries is the same. DAR denotes:

- Problem assessment **d**ata
- Nursing **a**ctions
- Evaluation of **r**esponses

SOAPIER denotes:

- **S**ubjective and **O**bjective data
- **A**ssessments
- **P**lan
- **I**ntervention strategies
- **E**valuations
- **R**evisions

How to Document: Basic Criteria

Good documentation is concise, accurate, complete, legible, timely, and logically organized. These criteria must be applied each time the nurse makes an entry on patient records.[5]

Accuracy of Patient Name, Dates, and Times

Each time patient data is recorded, the date and time must be included. Check to ensure that the patient's name is on all sheets on which you are recording information. For the same problems, be sure that the dates and times on the flow sheets match the dates and times in the progress notes.

A 24-hour clock, often referred to as *military time,* is used in most health-care facilities to clearly distinguish a.m. from p.m. hours (Table 7.1).

Accuracy of Entries

Always use objective and measurable terms about the patient's behaviors and speech. Objective data, also called *empirical sensory data,* include things you hear, see, feel, or smell. This information is strictly factual; it is not appropriate to write opinions, biased statements, or speculations. For example, if you are biased and label the patient "a complainer," you may miss important assessment information. Instead, write a quote about what the patient stated. Write only what you see, and let the reader draw conclusions. Remember, the patients have the right to read their charts at any time.

Table 7.1 **24-Hour Clock**	
1 p.m. = 1300	1 a.m. = 0100
2 p.m. = 1400	2 a.m. = 0200
3 p.m. = 1500	3 a.m. = 0300
4 p.m. = 1600	4 a.m. = 0400
5 p.m. = 1700	5 a.m. = 0500
6 p.m. = 1800	6 a.m. = 0600
7 p.m. = 1900	7 a.m. = 0700
8 p.m. = 2000	8 a.m. = 0800
9 p.m. = 2100	9 a.m. = 0900
10 p.m. = 2200	10 a.m. = 1000
11 p.m. = 2300	11 a.m. = 1100
12 midnight = 2400	12 noon = 1200

Legibility

All entries must be legible and in black ink. Write neatly, spell correctly, and write on the lines provided. Ink is used because it cannot be erased and can be photocopied. Illegible writing can lead to life-threatening situations that may be the result of medication or therapy errors. Always question and clarify illegible writing to avoid patient-care errors. Illegible medication and therapy orders are especially dangerous. In addition, start entries with a capital letter and end with a period.

Signatures

Always sign the document carefully, using the first letter of your name, your last name, and your title. Traditionally, SN has been the abbreviation for student nurse, LPN for licensed practical nurse, and RN for registered nurse. Because many nursing schools may share the same facility, you will be required to write the abbreviation of your school affiliation along with the title SN; for example: N. DiRenzo, YSU, SN.

Never sign anyone else's entry. You are accountable for whatever you sign. The only exception is if a caregiver has left the health-care agency for the day and calls in with information she forgot to document. Then the conversation must be documented in the progress notes, and corrections must be made on the records.

Correcting Mistakes

When you make a mistake, draw a single line through the words, write the word *error* above the mistaken words, and sign your name or initials. Then make the right entry. Always correct documentation errors promptly in order to avoid patient-care errors. Never erase entries; never use correction fluid, or never scribble out errors. It should not look like data was hidden or tampered with in any way.

Logical Organization of Information

To ensure correct sequencing of events, document on the standardized forms and progress notes as you go throughout the day. Do not wait until the end of the day to record what happened with patients. It is much easier to accurately re-member the sequence of events if you record them shortly after they occur. Also, do not docu-ment in advance. Other health-care providers are dependent on information you document to im-plement their plans of care, and there is potential for patient-care errors when documentation is not timely or accurate.

Always record data consecutively, line by line, in the progress notes. Never leave blank spaces in progress notes. If you leave blank spaces, another health-care provider can add in-correct information to the spaces. If space is left after you sign and date an entry, draw a line out to the right margin of the line.

Writing a Late Entry

Sometimes a nurse may forget to write some pa-tient data that needs to be included. Start the late entry with the current month, date, and time, and then write, "Addendum to nurse's note of __(month)/__(date)/___ (time)." Never try to squeeze in additional notes near previously writ-ten notes; always make addenda when you forget to enter information. A well-known rule of thumb to guide documentation is: "If you didn't record it, it wasn't done."

Completeness

All standardized forms must be filled out com-pletely, with spaces filled in with "not applicable" (NA) if it does not apply to the patient. For exam-ple, the menstrual cycle information is not appli-cable for male patients, and the blank would be filled in with NA.

Overgeneralizations can also be problematic. Specific information is needed. For example, what does "not having a good day" mean? Overgeneralizations waste space, lack objectivity, and are incomplete.

Omitted Strategies

Sometimes strategies are purposely omitted be-cause of the patient's condition or unavailability of the patient. For example, the patient has a daily laxative scheduled as a routine medication, but the patient now reports loose stools, so the nurse does not give the medication. The reason the drug is not given must be included in a progress note, and an order must be obtained from the physician to discontinue the drug. Sometimes the patient may be off the unit when the drugs are supposed to be given, so drugs are not given on time; a note must be made for why the drugs were not given at the specified time. Omissions without explanations are considered errors, be-cause, legally, you must do all you are supposed to do or give an explanation for why something is not done, and then notify the appropriate members of the health-care team.

Conciseness

Patient record entries must be brief, using incom-plete sentences. Eliminate all words that do not change the intended meaning of the entry, includ-ing articles such as "a" and "the," and also the subject of the sentence. Use standard abbrevia-tions for conciseness, but only those that are ap-proved by the health-care agency. You can concisely write patient or family comments, but you must put quotes around the actual words the patient spoke. The sample documentations previ-ously listed are examples of concise entries. Note that neither the patient's name nor the word "pa-tient" was written, because all entries are about the patient. Also, it is a waste of time and space to repeat in a narrative statement in the progress notes what was sufficiently covered on standard-ized forms.

Confidentiality

Patient privacy has always been an important part of nursing responsibilities. Patient informa-tion must be kept confidential and documenta-tion systems must be secure. The Health Insurance Portability and Accountability Act (HIPAA) was established to protect patient pri-vacy in written and electronic documentation. This 1996 legislation maintains the security of protected health information about patients. Be-fore the passage of this act, many patients did not know that their medical records could be released to other parties, such as insurance com-panies, employers, or researchers, without per-mission from patients. Nurses have always been advocates for patients' privacy, and now there are specific laws to protect privacy.[6]

Documentation of Communication With Physicians and Other Health-Care Providers

The Joint Commission has reported that communication errors are the root cause of 70% of sentinel events.[7] Sentinel events are defined as those resulting in serious physical or psychological injury, or death. Nurses must learn to give concise and informative verbal reports to physicians. Nurses are sometimes afraid to call certain physicians because they fear they will be reprimanded for being ill-timed or uninformative. Physicians complain about nurses calling inappropriately, and nurses complain about rude, disruptive behavior from physicians during telephone conversations. Nurses may delay care because they are afraid to call physicians. The style of nursing communication is often broad and narrative, when physicians are interested in a brief succinct report.

The communication problem has resulted in the development of the SBAR shared communication, model for nurses to use when giving telephone reports to physicians.[8] SBAR stands for *Situation-Background-Assessment-Recommendation*. The concept care map contains all the information that is needed for the SBAR tool. The Institute for Healthcare Improvement provides guidelines for communicating with physicians using the SBAR process, which are located in Box 7.1. This box provides a step-by-step guide for what to say as you give a patient report to a physician. The template for the SBAR report to a physician about a critical situation is located in Figure 7.6.

Whether in person or in a phone conversation, document discussions of patient care with other health-care providers. To decrease errors in communication, you can use your concept map to organize the SBAR report of what you will say over the phone to the physician. You must record what was discussed and what was done after the conversation. For example:

> *8/8/15 1500 Pain r/t incision: Dr. Morrow notified per phone Percodan (oxycodone/aspirin) did not relieve pain after 1 hour. States pain is "9" on 10-point scale. N. DiRenzo, YSU, SN*
>
> *1510 Per order, given 50 mg Demerol IM stat. See MAR [medication administration record]. N. DiRenzo, YSU, SN*
>
> *1545 Reports pain "4" on 10-point scale. States "pain much better, but still not gone." N. DiRenzo, YSU, SN*

Never write critical comments about another health-care provider or make entries suggesting an error or unsafe practice. For example, "Physician made error in the orders." Instead, write "Physician called to clarify order." It is standard practice to include in the written statement the objective patient behaviors that relate to the error or unsafe practice if applicable.

In the progress notes, always chart changes in the patient's condition, abnormal test results, and the time that the changes were reported to the physician. Additionally, report threats of legal action or bodily harm from the patient or family toward any member of the health-care team or organization. Record and report to the physician and hospital administrators when the patient displays risks to himself, such as drug or alcohol abuse, or if the patient is refusing treatment or is unwilling to comply with recommendations. Equipment malfunction is also recorded and reported to supervisors.

Box 7.1   GUIDELINES FOR COMMUNICATING WITH PHYSICIANS USING THE SBAR PROCESS

1. Use the following modalities according to the physician's preference, if known. Wait no longer than 5 minutes between attempts.
   - Direct page (if known)
   - Call service
   - During weekdays, the physician's office directly
   - On weekends and after hours during the week, physician's home phone
   - Cell phone

   Before assuming that the physician you are attempting to reach is not responding, utilize all modalities. For emergent situations, use appropriate resident service as needed to ensure safe patient care.

2. Prior to calling the physician, follow these steps:
   - Have I seen and assessed the patient myself before calling?
   - Has the situation been discussed with a resource nurse or preceptor?
   - Review the chart for the appropriate physician to call.
   - Know the admitting diagnosis and date of admission.
   - Have I read the most recent MD progress notes and notes from the nurse who worked the shift ahead of me?
   - Have available the following when speaking with the physician:
   - Patient's chart;
   - List of current medications, allergies, IV fluids, and laboratory results;
   - Most recent vital signs;
   - Code Status

When reporting laboratory results, provide the date and time and have ready the results of previous tests for comparison.

3. When calling the physician, follow the SBAR process:
   Situation: What is the situation you are calling about?
   - Identify self, unit, patient, room number.
   - Briefly state the problem—what it is, when it happened or started, and how severe it is.
   Background: Pertinent background information related to the situation could include the following:
   - The admitting diagnosis and date of admission
   - A list of current medications, allergies, IV fluids, and laboratory test results
   - Most recent vital signs
   - The date and time of any laboratory tests, and the results of previous tests for comparison
   - Other clinical information
   - Code status
   Assessment: What is the nurse's assessment of the situation?
   Recommendation: What is the nurse's recommendation or what does he/she want?

Examples:
   - Notification that the patient has been admitted
   - The patient needs to be seen now
   - Order change

4. Document the change in the patient's condition and physician notification.

Source: Kaiser Permanente SBAR Technique for Communication: A Situational Briefing Model © Kaiser Foundation Health Plan Inc., available at http://www.ihi.org, with permission.

S	**Situation** **I am calling about** \<patient's name and location\> **The patient's code status is** \<code status\> **The problem I am calling about is** —————————————————. 　　　　I am afraid the patient is going to arrest. **I have just assessed the patient personally:** **Vital signs are:** Blood pressure ——/——, Pulse——, Respiration——, and temperature—— **I am concerned about the:** 　　　　Blood pressure because it is over 200 or less than 100 or 30 mmHg below usual 　　　　Pulse because it is over 140 or less than 50 　　　　Respiration because it is less than 5 or over 40 　　　　Temperature because it is less than 96 or over 104
B	**Background** **The patient's mental status is:** 　　　　Alert and oriented to person place and time 　　　　Confused and cooperative or non-cooperative 　　　　Agitated or combative 　　　　Lethargic but conversant and able to swallow 　　　　Stuporous and not talking clearly and possibly not able to swallow 　　　　Comatose. Eyes closed. Not responding to stimulation. **The skin is:** 　　　　Warm and dry 　　　　Pale 　　　　Mottled 　　　　Diaphoretic 　　　　Extremities are cold 　　　　Extremities are warm **The patient is not or is on oxygen.** 　　　　The patient has been on —————— (l/min) or (%) oxygen for —————— minutes (hours) 　　　　The oximeter is reading ——% 　　　　The oximeter does not detect a good pulse and is giving erratic readings
A	**Assessment** 　　　　**This is what I think the problem is:** \<say what you think is the problem\> 　　　　**The problem seems to be cardiac infection neurologic respiratory**—————— 　　　　**I am not sure what the problem is but the patient is deteriorating.** 　　　　**The patient seems to be unstable and may get worse, we need to do something.**
R	**Recommendation** **I suggest or request that you** \<say what you would like to see done\>. 　　　　Transfer the patient to critical care. 　　　　Come to see the patient at this time. 　　　　Talk to the patient or family about code status. 　　　　Ask the on-call family practice resident to see the patient now. 　　　　Ask for a consultant to see the patient now. **Are any tests needed:** 　　　　Do you need any test like CXR, ABG, EKG, CBC, or BMP? 　　　　Other? **If a change in treatment is ordered, then ask:** 　　　　How often do you want vital signs? 　　　　How long do you expect this problem will last? 　　　　If the patient does not get better, when would you want us to call again?

● Figure 7.6   SBAR report to a physician. (Kaiser Permanente SBAR Technique for Communication: A Situational Briefing Model © Kaiser Foundation Health Plan Inc., available at http://www.ihi.org, with permission.)

CHAPTER 7 SUMMARY

Concept care maps are valuable guides for documentation of patient care. Documentation is very important, because it is the legal record of patient care, and in many instances the basis for financial reimbursement by insurance companies, Medicare, and Medicaid. Good documentation is concise, accurate, complete, legible, timely, logically organized, and confidential. It is a challenge to learn to document well, but concept care maps will help to remind you of all that must be documented. As the basis of documentation, you will use the diagram, outcomes, and strategies, as well as data collected regarding patient responses to strategies to complete standardized forms and narrative notes.

Routine assessments are performed and documented using standardized forms, with specific problems expanded upon in narrative form using progress notes. The progress notes include documentation of the patient's problems, nursing strategies and actions to correct the problems, and evaluation of patient responses to the nursing strategies. You must describe the problem succinctly, describe what you did about the problem, and then describe the patient response to the nursing strategies you did to alleviate the problem.

Documentation of communication with other health-care providers is extremely important to avoid patient care errors. The concept care map can be used to guide the development of the SBAR to improve the succinct and accurate report to a physician and decrease sentinel events.

LEARNING ACTIVITIES

1. The following are charting excerpts taken from actual medical records. For each entry, what needs to be done to correct it?
   - *By the time he was admitted, his rapid heart had stopped, and he was feeling better.*
   - *Patient has chest pain if she lies on her left side for over a year.*
   - *She has had no rigors or shaking chills, but her husband says she was very hot in bed last night.*
   - *The patient has been depressed since she began seeing me in 1993.*
   - *I have suggested that he loosen his pants before standing, and then, he stands with the help of his wife, they should fall to the floor.*
   - *Healthy appearing decrepit 69-year-old male, mentally alert but forgetful.*
   - *Patient has left his white blood cells at another hospital.*
   - *The patient refused an autopsy.*
   - *The patient is tearful and crying constantly. She also appears to be depressed.*
   - *Large brown stool ambulating in the hall.*
   - *Skin: somewhat pale but present.*
   - *Patient has two teenage children but no other abnormalities.*
   - *The patient had waffles for breakfast and anorexia for lunch.*
   - *She slipped on ice and her legs went in separate directions in early December.*
   - *Discharge status: Alive but without permission.*
   - *Patient released to the outpatient department without dressing.*
   - *The patient expired on the floor uneventfully.*
   - *The patient has no past history of suicides.*
   - *Since she can't get pregnant without her husband, I thought you would like to work her up.*
   - *The patient will need disposition, and therefore we will get Dr. Smith to dispose of him.*

2. Practice writing narrative progress notes for the concept care map of the diabetic patient from the case studies in previous chapters. Use Figures 5.1 and 5.2 from Chapter 5.

3. Practice using the concept care map in Figures 5.1 and 5.2 to develop an SBAR.

REFERENCES

1. *Nursing: Scope and Standards of Practice*. 2nd ed. Silver Spring, Md: American Nurses Association; 2010.

2. *2014 Comprehensive Accreditation Manual for Hospitals: The Official Handbook*. Chicago, Ill: The Joint Commission; 2014.

3. Charting Tips: Easy as PIE. *Nursing99*. 1999;29(4):25. (seminal article)

4. Springhouse Publishing Company Staff. *Documentation in Action*. Philadelphia, Pa: Lippincott, Williams and Wilkins; 2005.

5. *ANA's Principles for Nursing Documentation*. Silver Spring, Md: American Nurses Association; 2010.

6. U.S. Department of Health and Human Services. *Health Information Privacy*. Available at: http://www.hhs.gov/ocr/ privacy. Last Accessed September 14, 2014.

7. The Joint Commission. Sentinel Event Data: Root Causes by Event Type. Available at: http://www.jointcommission.org/ assets/1/18/Root_Causes_by_Event_ Type_2004-2Q2013.pdf . Last Accessed September 14, 2014.

8. Institute for Healthcare Improvement. SBAR technique for communication: a situational briefing model. Available at: http://ihi.org/IHI/Topics/PatientSafety/ SafetyGeneral/Tools/SBARTechniquefor-CommunicationASituationalBriefing-Model.htm. Last Accessed September 14, 2014.

AFTER THE CLINICAL DAY IS OVER: PATIENT EVALUATIONS, SELF-EVALUATIONS, AND GRADING THE FINAL CONCEPT CARE MAP

1. Identify standards of professional performance related to patient care evaluations and performance evaluations.

2. Describe the purposes of performance evaluations.

3. Compare formative and summative evaluations.

4. Explain what to do when an error is made.

5. Compare constructive criticism with negative criticism.

6. Analyze criteria for dismissal from clinical.

7. Identify criteria for grading concept care maps.

The clinical day is over, and there is very little left to do. Students spend only about 30 to 60 minutes after leaving the clinical site summarizing patient progress toward goals and outcome objectives and performing self-evaluations of their clinical performance. The time is spent reflecting on clinical performance and patient responses to nursing strategies, and writing summaries. The primary focus of this chapter is on professional nursing performance during the clinical day. The American Nurses Association (ANA) has developed Standards of Professional Performance. The registered nurse is responsible for evaluation of the effectiveness of his or her own practice in relation to professional practice standards and guidelines and state practice laws.[1]

A very important aspect of a nurse's professional responsibility is a self-evaluation of performance. Your self-evaluation must be an accurate perception of your abilities. Your clinical faculty will also evaluate your performance weekly, with periodic summary evaluations.

In addition to performing a self-evaluation, you will need to finish evaluation of patient responses and patient progress toward objectives, which you started earlier at the clinical site. Analyze and record patients' physical and emotional behavioral responses. Evaluate the extent to which the patient objectives were attained or not, and write about it under the evaluation summary of the patient progress toward the outcome objectives, as described in Chapter 5.

This chapter also provides criteria for grading the concept care map. You need to know the criteria that will be used for grading the concept care map so that you can earn an A on your final edition of the concept care map.

Purpose of Performance Evaluations

A performance evaluation is the process of determining how well the nursing student does what is required. Both you and your clinical faculty will evaluate your performance. As the faculty critiques your performance, the purpose is not to blame or shame students. The questions to be addressed in the performance evaluation are: Do you provide safe and effective care? What grade did you earn? By the end of the term, should you be promoted to the next level?[2-4]

Your performance will be compared to established standards that define goals to be attained over time. Each course has expected performance standards that will be stated very clearly and in measurable behaviors. The clinical objectives and specific daily objectives of the course are used as standards to evaluate performance. Performance evaluations are based on those standards and objective criteria, not on personalities or whether a faculty member likes a student. Students must "own" and accept the consequences of their mistakes. Sometimes mistakes lead to a bad grade on a test in a theory course; sometimes they lead to poor patient care or accidental injury to a student. The following

are sample objectives for clinical evaluations, categorized by nursing process, documentation, and professional qualities.

Clinical Performance Objectives

Identify your strengths and weaknesses for each of the following clinical objectives:

Assessment

1. Prepares each patient profile by gathering complete, relevant information needed to develop a concept care map.
   a. Defines medical diagnoses
   b. Defines surgical procedures and diagnostic tests
   c. Defines diagnostic test reports
   d. Defines treatments
   e. Defines medications
   f. Obtains health assessment data from the records

Nursing Diagnoses

1. Develops a concept care map diagram.
   a. Identifies physiological, psychological, and educational problems
   b. Prioritizes diagnoses
   c. Correctly categorizes data on the map
   d. Correctly links diagnoses

Planning

1. Develops patient goals, objectives, and nursing strategies.
   a. Lists goals and objectives for each diagnosis
   b. Lists nursing strategies to attain objectives
   c. States rationales for strategies

Implementation

1. Provides safe and effective nursing care.
   a. Obtains change of shift information and integrates on care map
   b. Checks for updated orders at the beginning of the day and throughout the day and integrates on the care map

c. Organizes time, works in an organized manner, and gets care completed on time

d. Immediately reports assessment abnormalities and problems to the clinical faculty or to a staff nurse

e. Keeps bed down and locked, with side rails up, and call light within patient's reach when not with the patient

f. Maintains a safe environment by avoiding activities that could potentially put self or others at risk for injury and by using correct protective strategies for patients, coworkers, and self

g. Leaves patient's room neat and clean

h. Continually checks patient's safety and comfort needs throughout clinical day

2. Safely and effectively implements all procedures and treatments.

a. Practices and reviews procedures and treatments prior to clinical

b. Determines basic-care needs and safely performs all procedures without being reminded (examples: cough and deep breath, turning, intake and output, range of motion, vital signs, skin care)

c. Follows standard precautions with all procedures and treatments

d. Follows hospital and departmental policies with all procedures and treatments

e. Displays confidence and composure when carrying out procedures and treatments

f. Prepares patient/family prior to procedures/treatments

g. Shows respect for privacy needs

h. Involves family in care of patient

3. Safely and effectively administers medications.

a. Rechecks the medication records each morning for updates

b. Questions discrepancies in medication records

c. Checks for medication allergies on chart and patient armband

d. Demonstrates knowledge of medications

e. Accurately calculates medication doses with 100% accuracy

f. Accurately calculates intravenous flow rates

g. Assesses the six rights prior to administering any medication

h. Checks appropriate laboratory work related to medication administration

i. Evaluates assessment data prior to medication administration

j. Checks all medications with faculty prior to administration

k. Uses proper technique when preparing and administering medications

l. Gives all medications in the allotted time period

4. Safely and effectively teaches, and is emotionally supportive to, patients and families.

a. Uses the METHOD teaching plan

b. Provides teaching for patients and family as needed related to METHOD

c. Demonstrates knowledge of teaching-learning and developmental principles

d. Answers patient/family's questions and gives explanations in appropriate and understandable terms without causing the patient or family undue anxiety

e. Provides psychosocial and cultural support for patient and families, including the use of touch, humor, empathy, anticipatory guidance, play, relaxation techniques, distraction, reminiscence, and music

5. Communicates effectively.

a. Demonstrates appropriate verbal and nonverbal behaviors in patient/family care

b. Avoids saying or doing anything that could cause undue anxiety for the patient or family

c. Reports off to the faculty and appropriate personnel when leaving for breaks or at the end of clinical

d. Communicates as needed with other health-care providers in planning and carrying out the plan of care

e. Informs the faculty and cover nurse immediately of any changes in the patient's condition or when any problem is encountered

f. Is pleasant and courteous during all interactions, using professional communication strategies
6. Collaborates with other health-care workers.
   a. Actively participates as a health-care team member
   b. Discusses care planning with others (faculty, students, staff)
   c. Assists other patients at the site in addition to those assigned
   d. Interacts effectively with faculty, students, and staff to accomplish objectives
   e. Assists other health-care team members as time permits
   f. Actively participates in preconferences and postconferences

Evaluation

1. Evaluates the concept care map.
   a. Assesses the patient's progress toward objectives
   b. Assesses patient's behavioral responses to nursing strategies
   c. Modifies the plan of care, as needed, based on reassessment
2. Evaluates self-performance.
   a. Objectively assesses self-performance
   b. Immediately admits mistakes and takes actions to correct them
   c. Accepts constructive criticism without making excuses for behaviors
   d. Assumes responsibility for own actions; knows limitations and when to seek guidance
   e. Performs weekly, midterm, and final self-evaluations
   f. Identifies own strengths and weaknesses
   g. Sets own goals and objectives and strives to attain them
   h. Seeks appropriate experiences at agencies to meet individual needs

Documentation

1. Documents accurately, concisely, completely, and in a timely manner.

a. Records assessment data on appropriate forms (such as flow sheets or progress notes)
b. Documents without being reminded
c. Consults faculty when recording abnormal assessment findings
d. Demonstrates neatness and organization of writing on patient records; uses correct terminology, phraseology, and spelling
e. Follows agency policy regarding documentation (such as using approved abbreviations and black ink only) and corrects errors in charting with one line

Professional Qualities

1. Acts professionally at all times.
   a. Follows ANA Standards of Practice and Standards of Professional Performance at all times
   b. Follows all policies of the nursing program regarding clinical conduct
   c. Updates CPR certification, immunizations, and tuberculosis test yearly
   d. Follows the dress code, presenting with professional attire and behavior during clinical and when obtaining assignments
   e. Submits written work that is neat, organized, complete, and on time
   f. Carefully follows directions
   g. Takes the initiative in arranging for make-up of missed written or clinical work
   h. Is punctual in reporting to or leaving the clinical agency; when ill, calls the agency and faculty prior to scheduled arrival time
2. Acts ethically at all times.
   a. Shows respect for patient and family
   b. Calls patient by name and title
   c. Respects patient's personal space
   d. Maintains confidentiality related to patient information
   e. Follows ANA Code of Ethics for Nurses

Your clinical faculty will use critical incidents, rating scales, or both to help you identify your strengths and weaknesses. Weekly clinical performance appraisal recordings are used to document actual incidents of successful or unsuccessful performance. In using the critical incident approach, you will be asked to list specific actions, reactions, or attributes that were strengths or weaknesses. Two sample clinical performance appraisal assessment forms are shown in Figures 8.1 and 8.2. Faculty will specify the specific behaviors that are expected, dependent on course objectives. In Figure 8.1, note that you must complete an accurate self-evaluation, and that faculty comments are next to yours. Figure 8.2 is a sample anecdotal note that is completed when a student's performance is not acceptable; the clinical situation is carefully documented, and the anecdotal note may be placed in the student's academic record.

Constructive Criticism

Criticism is a fact of life and something we all must face. The only way to avoid criticism is to live isolated from other people, but a career in nursing is anything but isolated. We all have had our work, our personalities, and our behaviors criticized at some point. No matter how hard we try, someone is going to be unhappy with us about something; actually, the best any of us can do is to please some of the people some of the time. Sometimes criticism is ungrounded and is based on a difference of opinion.[5] In this case, one opinion is as good as any other, provided you believe in respecting others' rights to their opinions. In this situation, be assertive and say, "Your opinion is noted. However, I do not agree and plan to continue etc."

Other times, the criticism received is valuable and helpful and thus requires changing behaviors. The valuable and helpful criticism is termed *constructive criticism*. Faculty use constructive criticism to correct and guide student performance in clinical settings. Its intent is not to shame or blame on a personal level; the intent of constructive criticism from your nursing faculty is to give you feedback on your performance and to help you grow into your role as a professional nurse.

Carrying Out Responsibilities and Showing Initiative

As a nursing student, you have many responsibilities, that grow with each term in the nursing program. You are expected to perform to the best of your ability and also to take the initiative and look for opportunities to learn new information and skills. For whatever level in nursing you are currently in, there will be specific skills to perform and specific methods to use in performing them. Once you know your responsibilities, it is up to you to carry them out. If you are unsure of what to do or are afraid of not doing something well, consult with your clinical faculty to get some help. If you do not know how to do something, ask. It is better to admit that you do not know something than to have your clinical faculty find out when something is not done. The latter scenario would reflect poorly on you and—more seriously—may jeopardize patient safety.

The fastest way to be dismissed from clinical and possibly even from the nursing program is to jeopardize patient safety. Performance appraisals are used to decide if a student should be dismissed. Not everyone has the ability to be a nurse. Following are some samples of unacceptable clinical behaviors, taken from the Youngstown State University Department of Nursing Undergraduate Student Handbook[6].

Dismissal for Unacceptable Clinical Behavior Policy

The Department of Nursing reserves the right to dismiss a student from the program and/or clinical who demonstrates unacceptable clinical behaviors that include, but are not limited to:

1. Failure to pick up a clinical assignment or inadequate preparation for clinical experience;
2. Attending clinical experiences under the influence of drugs and/or alcohol;
3. Refusing to care for an assigned patient based on patient's characteristics; e.g., race, culture, religious beliefs, or diagnosis;
4. Participating in acts of omission or commission in the care of patients, such as physical abuse; placing the patient in a

WEEKLY CLINICAL SELF EVALUATION   Student _____

Date of Clinical _____

Patient Initials: _____ Age: ____ Medical Diagnosis(es) _____

Allergies: _____

	Faculty Comments
ASSESSMENT–Prepares each patient profile by gathering complete information needed to develop a care map. Describe medical diagnoses, surgical procedures, diagnostic tests, treatments, medications, physical assessment data. **STUDENT COMMENTS** YOUR STRENGTHS: YOUR WEAKNESSES AND REMEDY TO IMPROVE:	
NURSING DIAGNOSIS(ES)–Brings to clinical each week a concept care map and identifies physiological and psycho-social problems, correctly categorizes data on the map, prioritizes problems, links problems and labels diagnoses. **STUDENT COMMENTS** YOUR STRENGTHS: YOUR WEAKNESSES AND REMEDY TO IMPROVE:	
PLANNING–Comes prepared to clinical with a developed care map that include goals, objectives, and strategies; and states rationales for nursing strategies. Collaborates with staff, faculty, and students in planning coordinated nursing care. Participates in clincal pre and post conferences. **STUDENT COMMENTS** YOUR STRENGTHS: YOUR WEAKNESSES AND REMEDY TO IMPROVE:	
IMPLEMENTATION Safely performs procedures and medication administration. Organizes time, works in an organized manner, and gets care completed on time. Uses therapeutic communication techniques such as touch, humor, empathy, anticipatory guidance, relaxation techniques, distraction, reminiscence, and music to reduce anxiety. Interacts effectively with staff, faculty, and other students. **STUDENT COMMENTS** YOUR STRENGTHS: YOUR WEAKNESSES AND REMEDY TO IMPROVE:	
Patient EVALUATION: Assesses patient's progress toward objectives and responses to nursing strategies and modifies the plan as needed. Informs the faculty and cover nurse immediately regarding any changes in the patient condition or when any problem is encountered. **STUDENT COMMENTS** YOUR STRENGTHS: YOUR WEAKNESSES AND REMEDY TO IMPROVE:	
Self-EVALUATION: Admits mistakes and takes actions to correct them, accepts constructive criticism, seeks out experiences, knows limitations, and seeks guidance when needed. **STUDENT COMMENTS** YOUR STRENGTHS: YOUR WEAKNESSES AND REMEDY TO IMPROVE:	
DOCUMENTATION: Documents accurately, concisely, completely, and in a timely manner. Consults faculty before documenting abnormal findings. Follows agency policies regarding documentation. **STUDENT COMMENTS** YOUR STRENGTHS: YOUR WEAKNESSES AND REMEDY TO IMPROVE:	
PROFESSIONAL QUALITIES: Follows ANA standards of care and code of ethics, follows the dress codes and all policies of the nursing program regarding clinical conduct. Is always on time and comes with prepared care plan. **STUDENT COMMENTS** YOUR STRENGTHS: YOUR WEAKNESSES AND REMEDY TO IMPROVE:	

● Figure 8.1   Hospital weekly objectives, clinical self-evaluation, and faculty evaluation.

Youngstown State University
Bachelor Degree Program in Nursing

Nursing _____ – _____

Semester, 20 ____

Anecdotal Note

Name of Student: _____ Date: _____

The Situation

_____
_____
_____
_____

Description of Student's Actions

_____
_____
_____
_____

Instructor's Evaluation

_____
_____
_____
_____

Instructor's Signature: _____

● Figure 8.2 **Anecdotal note.**

hazardous position, condition, or circumstance; mental/emotional abuse;

5. Disrupting of patient care or unit functioning related to poor interpersonal relationships with agency health team members, peers, or faculty;

6. Demonstrating behavior that affects one or more parameters of safe clinical practice and/or jeopardizes the well-being of the patient, patient families, health team members, peers, or faculty;

7. Documenting dishonestly, breaching patient confidentiality, solicitation of patient for services leading to personal gain, and other behaviors as listed under Professionalism Category of the Clinical Evaluation Tool.

8. Failing to adhere to the Ohio Board of Nursing Rules Regulating the Practice of Nursing as of February 1, 2009, 4723-5-12.
   ▶ A student shall report and document nursing assessments or observations,

the care provided by the student for the patient, and the patient's response to that care;

▶ A student shall accurately and timely report to the appropriate practitioner errors in or deviations from the prescribed regimen of care;

▶ A student shall not falsify any patient record or any other document prepared or utilized in the course of, or in conjunction with, nursing practice;

▶ A student shall implement measures to promote a safe environment for each patient;

▶ A student shall delineate, establish, and maintain professional boundaries with each patient;

▶ At all times when a student is providing direct nursing care to a patient the student shall:

(a) Provide privacy during examination or treatment and in the care of personal or bodily needs; and

(b) Treat each patient with courtesy, respect, and with full recognition of dignity and individuality;

▶ A student shall not:

(a) Engage in behavior that causes or may cause physical, verbal, mental, or emotional abuse to a patient; or

(b) Engage in behavior toward a patient that may reasonably be interpreted as physical, verbal, mental, or emotional abuse;

▶ A student shall not misappropriate a patient's property or:

(a) Engage in behavior to seek or obtain personal gain at the patient's expense;

(b) Engage in behavior that may reasonably be interpreted as behavior to seek or obtain personal gain at the patient's expense;

(c) Engage in behavior that constitutes inappropriate involvement in the patient's personal relationships; or

(d) Engage in behavior that may reasonably be interpreted as inappropriate involvement in the patient's personal relationships;

For the purpose of the above paragraph, the patient is always presumed incapable of giving free, full, or informed consent to the behaviors by the student set forth in this paragraph.

▶ A student shall not:

(a) Engage in sexual conduct with a patient;

(b) Engage in conduct that may reasonably be interpreted as sexual;

(c) Engage in any verbal behavior that is seductive or sexually demeaning to a patient; or

(d) Engage in verbal behavior that may reasonably be interpreted as seductive or sexually demeaning to a patient;

For the purpose of the above paragraph, the patient is always presumed incapable of giving free, full, or informed consent to sexual activity with the student.

The student's behavior must demonstrate competency by responsible preparation, implementation, and documentation of the nursing care of patients. In addition, the student's behavior must be respectful of all individuals (patient, patient's family, health team members, and self) according to the American Hospital Association A Patient's Bill of Rights, the ANA Standards of Practice, and the ANA Code of Ethics for Nurses.

Due Process

A student who exhibits unacceptable clinical behavior and/or violates student conduct requirements set forth by the Ohio Board of Nursing will be given a verbal and written performance report by the clinical faculty member. The performance report becomes part of the student's academic record.

The faculty member will notify the Admission Progression and Graduation (AP&G) Committee of the student's conduct, violation, and/or unacceptable behavior for further consideration. The AP&G Committee will consider documented evidence from the student, faculty, or health-care team members when making recommendations regarding continuation of the student's participation in the program and/or clinical. The AP&G Committee recommendation will be presented to the General Faculty and/or Chairperson of the Department of Nursing for the final decision. The student will be notified of the decision, in writing, by the AP&G Committee.

Clinical Evaluations: Formative and Summative

Clinical faculty expect students to be in a state of continuous development throughout the nursing program and to make increasing contributions to the clinical care of patients. There are links between performance evaluation, professional growth and development, and the rewards of providing excellent care.[7-9] Faculty and students give feedback to each other in order to evaluate the student's performance, professional growth, and development. The focus is on behaviors and skills. Students and faculty alike receive rewards when

the care of patients is done well. Faculty members are very proud of students who receive compliments from both the patients and the staff for the good job they are doing or have done, and students are proud of themselves. The cycle of performance, evaluation, professional growth, and reward is detailed in Figure 8.3.

Formative Evaluations

Start out each term by reviewing specific clinical objectives that you will need to meet in order to complete the course. It is very important for you to be aware of what is expected of you. Then, weekly, you and your faculty will jointly select experiences to meet those objectives. For example, during the term just completed, you did not have time to perfect your injection skills, so you ask your faculty to arrange some additional experiences to develop this skill while you work on attainment of current course objectives.

THE CYCLE OF PERFORMANCE, EVALUATION, PROFESSIONAL GROWTH, AND REWARDS

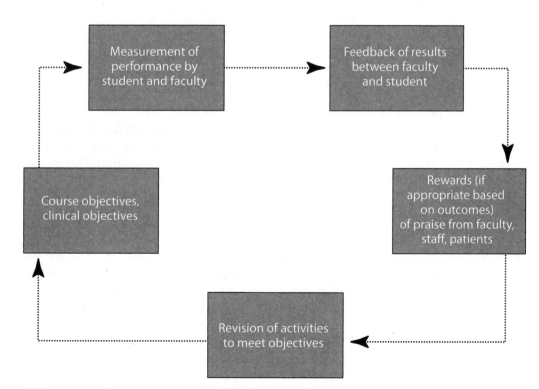

● Figure 8.3   The cycle of performance, evaluation, professional growth, and reward.

Weekly, there will be ongoing progress reviews and guidance from your clinical faculty. Students do weekly self-evaluations of strengths and weaknesses with regard to attaining the course objectives. You must objectively write down what you have done well or what needs improvement. Be sure to include any feedback from your faculty in your assessment. Faculty want to see that you remember what you were told during the clinical experience. When you give your self-evaluation to the faculty, they will write their comments. The intent is to monitor behaviors and skills closely, because human lives are at stake. It is very important that you know weekly what your clinical faculty member thinks of your performance.

Nurses have awesome responsibilities for the safe care of patients, and you and your faculty are working together very closely to prevent catastrophic mistakes from occurring. Faculty and students alike recognize that mistakes will be made, but avoiding a catastrophic mistake is the primary objective.

Summative Evaluations

Each clinical course also entails summative evaluations. Usually at midterm and at the end of the term, you and your clinical faculty will have a summative formal conference to review your progress toward meeting course objectives. At midterm, you and your faculty will establish individualized performance objectives for you to accomplish by the end of the term. With weekly formative evaluations, nothing at the summative review should come as a surprise. You and your faculty will review how you have done relative to the clinical objectives. If problems in attaining clinical objectives occur, there must be a discussion about why the objectives have not been met, and a new plan needs to be developed for meeting the objectives within the time constraints of the term. Specific steps are then decided upon that must be taken for improvement.

Whether the evaluation is formative or summative, there are some basic principles of receiving an evaluation to guide you:[9]

1. View all constructive criticism as having been given with helpful intent.
2. Listen to your faculty's perspective, and avoid excuses.
3. Ask for clarification, and for examples of any inappropriate behavior.
4. Check with your clinical faculty for mutual understanding.
5. Ask for help and support.

Now You've Blown It: Making Mistakes

Perhaps you recapped a contaminated needle, forgot to aspirate, or forgot to wear gloves when doing a subcutaneous injection and there was some bleeding at the site. Now what? First, remember that everyone makes mistakes, because no one is perfect. It is part of human nature to make mistakes. You must accept responsibility and be straightforward: "I really blew it by not aspirating." Admit your mistake; do not make excuses because doing so will indicate to your faculty that you cannot accept responsibility for what you have done. Here is a sample excuse from student to faculty: "You made me so nervous by being in the room with me that I forgot to aspirate." Your faculty does not want to listen to excuses, and will lose respect for you if you use them. Blaming your faculty for your lack of performance is certainly an avoidance of responsibility.

Suppose your clinical faculty was not there to see the mistake. For example, you neglect to get a patient up for ambulation in the morning because the patient said he was too weak to move. The staff nurse goes to assess the patient, asks him if he has walked yet, finds out he has not, and irately tells you that the patient must be walked immediately. Do you tell your faculty about it or not? Maybe the faculty member will not find out and you can cover it up. Honesty and integrity are paramount to safe and effective nursing care. It is much better for you to tell your faculty about your error in judgment than to let the clinical faculty find out about it from someone else. Faculty want to hear about the error from you directly, because it demonstrates that you take responsibility by owning up to your mistakes. If the faculty thinks that you are purposely covering up an error, it means that you cannot be trusted. A student covering up mistakes is acting dishonestly and unethically.

Second, do not beat yourself up about mistakes publicly or privately. It is unhealthy to engage in self-recrimination or statements such as "I'm stupid and will never make a good nurse." A better way to think is: "I'm intelligent, but I made a mistake that I will never make again." Focus on the behavior that you need to improve. You need to learn and grow from the mistake. Analyze what went wrong and do not repeat the error.[10]

Grading Concept Care Maps: How to Get an "A"

Figure 8.4 contains a sample care plan grading criteria form for the concept care map. For each criterion, one point is given if you do a good job summarizing information, a half of a point is given for some correct information with some information that is either incorrect or missing, and zero points are given if you have done a poor job on the information. This sample care plan criteria is useful for a medical-surgical hospitalized patient. Criteria will vary depending on the type of clinical setting and the level of the course in the curriculum. Good luck with concept care maps... it takes much time and effort to learn to organize and provide patient care, but your efforts will bring many satisfying rewards and you will become an excellent nurse!

CHAPTER 8 SUMMARY

You need ongoing exchanges with clinical faculty about performance for successful growth through constructive criticism and evaluation. Both the faculty and you sometimes need to say hard things, although in a respectful manner, by being open and honest, and you should trust each other to have your best interests in mind. Avoid becoming defensive or argumentative; stick with the facts. You will be receiving regular, constructive, and candid feedback from your clinical faculty. Your faculty will direct you where to go for assistance as needed (for example, the references to review or the skills laboratory for further practice, the mathematics center, or the writing center).

However, you alone must take responsibility for your own development. You must seek out learning experiences to develop yourself in ways that support the achievement of outstanding nursing care.

LEARNING ACTIVITIES

1. Compare course objectives from two sequential clinical nursing courses. Describe differences in focus and expectations.

2. Analyze clinical performance objectives for a nursing clinical experience, and give examples of behaviors that may be considered strengths and weaknesses.

3. Review your school's dismissal policy and compare it to the sample in the chapter.

4. Use the sample grading guide in Figure 8.4 to grade a concept care map you have developed.

ANA Standard I Assessment

General Survey	0 1/2 1
Health Assessment Data Base (Chapter 2)	0 1/2 1
Medical Diagnoses	0 1/2 1
Surgical Procedures	0 1/2 1
Medications	0 1/2 1
Laboratory	0 1/2 1
Skin Assessment Complete (Chapter 3)	0 1/2 1
Falls Assessment Complete (Chapter 3)	0 1/2 1
Glasgow Coma Scale (Chapter 3)	0 1/2 1
Psychosocial Assessment (Chapter 6)	0 1/2 1
Pain Assessment (Chapter 3)	0 1/2 1

ANA Standard 2 Diagnoses-Steps 1-3 Map-Chapter 3

Identifies Physiological Problems	0 1/2 1
Identifies Psychological Problems	0 1/2 1
Identifies Education Needs	0 1/2 1
Correctly Links Problems	0 1/2 1
Correctly Identifies Reason for Health Care (central box)	0 1/2 1
Key Assessments (central box)	0 1/2 1
Abnormal Assessment Data in correct boxes	0 1/2 1
Medications Categorized in correct boxes	0 1/2 1
Treatments Categorized in correct boxes	0 1/2 1
Diagnostic Tests in correct boxes	0 1/2 1
Correctly Prioritizes Problems	0 1/2 1
Correctly Labels Nursing Diagnoses (NANDA)	0 1/2 1

ANA Standards 3, 4 Outcomes, Planning-Steps 4 Chapter 4

Lists goals for all

Physical Problems	0 1/2 1
Psychosocial Problems	0 1/2 1

Lists objectives for all

Physical Problems	0 1/2 1
Psychosocial Problems	0 1/2 1

Lists all nursing strategies to attain objectives

Assessments to be Performed	0 1/2 1
Communication/Psychological Strategies	0 1/2 1
Physiological Strategies	0 1/2 1
Nursing strategies provide for patient/family participation	0 1/2 1

ANA Standard 6 Evaluation-Step 5 Chapter 5

Evaluates patients behavioral responses to nursing strategies for

1 Priority physical nursing diagnosis	0 1/2 1
1 Priority psychosocial nursing diagnosis	0 1/2 1

Under impressions, evaluate patient progress toward

Outcome objectives for

1 priority physical diagnosis	0 1/2 1
1 priority psychosocial diagnosis	0 1/2 1
Total Points	_/35 =_

● Figure 8.4   Sample evaluation form with grading criteria for a concept map care plan evaluation.

REFERENCES

1. *Nursing: Scope and Standards of Practice*. 2nd ed. Silver Spring, Md: American Nurses Association; 2010.

2. Gilmore S, Williams S. *Human Resource Management*. 2nd ed. New York, NY: Oxford University Press; 2013.

3. Pynes JE. *Human Resources Management for Public and Nonprofit Organizations*. 4th ed. San Francisco, Ca: Jossey-Bass Publishers; 2013.

4. Flynn WJ, Mathis RL, Jackson JH, Valentine S. *Healthcare Human Resource Management*. 3rd ed. Independence, Ky: Cengage Learning; 2015.

5. Carlson R. *Don't Sweat the Small Stuff at Work*. New York, NY: Hyperion; 1999.

6. Youngstown State University Department of Nursing Undergraduate Student Handbook, 2015.

7. Truss C, Mankin D, Kelliher C. *Strategic Human Resource Management*. New York, NY: Oxford University Press; 2012.

8. Carr C. *The New Manager's Survival Manual: All the Skills You Need for Success*. 2nd ed. New York, NY: John Wiley and Sons; 1995.

9. Mabey C, et al. *Human Resource Management: A Strategic Introduction*. 2nd ed. Malden, Mass: Blackwell; 1998.

10. Komisarjevsky C, Komisarjevsky R. *Peanut Butter and Jelly Management: Tales from Parenthood, Lessons for Managers*. New York, NY: American Management Association; 2003.

APPENDIX

Practice Case Studies

Assessment data for two patients, one surgical adult patient and one medical adult patient, have been provided in the Appendix. Review the data and use the concept map template (copy from the text or download the electronic version on DavisPlus) to create your concept map care plan.

1. Appendectomy – Surgical Patient (S. Lisko)
2. Osteoarthritis and Dementia – Medical Patient (M. Shortreed)

Additional practice case studies are listed below for Medical-Surgical as well as specialty patients – Psych, Critical Care, OB, and Pediatrics are available on DavisPlus at http://davispl.us/schuster4.

Medical-Surgical – Long Term Care Adult

1. Cancer of Lung with Lobectomy (P. Schuster)
2. Hip Fracture with Delayed Wound Healing, Osteoporosis (A. Weaver)

Medical-Surgical – Hospitalized Adult

1. Cerebral Vascular Accident with Aspiration Pneumonia (P. Schuster)
2. Orthostatic Hypotension, COPD (B. Thompson)
3. Arthroplasty of Right Hip, Osteoarthritis (B. Thompson)
4. Parkinson's Disease and Trauma Due to Falling (M. Roche)

Psych

1. Bipolar with Psychosis (K. Clark)
2. Depression with Polysubstance Abuse (M. Lukach)

Critical Care

1. Opioid Overdose with Renal Failure and Respiratory Depression (C. Shields)
2. Sleep Apnea with Respiratory Failure (C. Shields)

OB – Hospitalized Mother-Newborn

1. C-section and Gestational Diabetes (L. Aurilio)
2. Newborn with Jaundice (L. Aurilio)
3. Newborn of Mother with Gestational Diabetes (V. O'Dell)
4. Vaginal Delivery for Gravida 9 (S. Rendano)
5. Vaginal Delivery with Laceration and Repair (S. Rendano)

Pediatrics – Hospitalized Children

1. Cystic Fibrosis (N. Wagner, K. Serroka)
2. Osteosarcoma with Chemotherapy (J. Rankin)
3. Respiratory Syncytial Virus (K. Serroka, N. Wagner)
4. Sickle Cell Crisis (J. Rankin)
5. Tonsillectomy (N. Wagner)

Case Study: Appendectomy

1) Date of Care: 12/7/14	2) Patient Initials: PS	3) Age: 19	3) Growth and Development Intimacy Vs. Isolation	4) Gender: F	5) Admission Date: 12/6/14

6) Reason for hospitalization: Medical Dx: **Appendicitis** Pathophysiology: All signs and symptoms: **C/O periumbilical pain, vomiting, and diarrhea, low grade temperature, CAT scan showed inflamed appendix and elevated WBC's (18,000).**	7) Chronic illnesses: **None known**
8) Name of surgical procedure: **Appendectomy** Describe surgery: **General anesthesia, laparoscope, minimal blood loss—appendix adhered to abdominal wall and was dissected away from wall prior to removal.**	

9) ADVANCE DIRECTIVES (NURSE'S ADMISSION ASSESSMENTS):

Living will: ☐ Yes ☒ No	Power of attorney: ☐ Yes ☒ No	Do not resuscitate (DNR) order: ☐ Yes ☒ No

10) LABORATORY DATA:

Test	Normal Values	Admission	Date/Time	Date/Time	Reason for Abnormal Value
White blood cells (WBCs)		18.4			
Red blood cells (RBCs)					
Hemoglobin (Hgb)		14.1			
Hematocrit (Hct)		42			
Platelets					
Prothrombin time (PT)					
International normalized ratio (INR)					
Activated partial thromboplastin time (Aptt)					
Sodium Na		142			
Potassium K		4.6			
Chloride Cl		106			
Glucose (FBS/BS)		93			
CO_2		27			
Magnesium		2.2			
Calcium		10.1			
Hemoglobin A1C					
Cholesterol					
Blood Urea Nitrogen (BUN)					
Creatinine					
Urine analysis (UA)					
Pre-albumin					
Albumin					
Calcium Ca					
Phosphate					
Bilirubin					
Alkaline phosphatase					
SGOT-Serum glutamic-oxyloacetic transaminase					
AST-Serum glutamic pyruvic transaminase					
CK					
CK MB					
Troponin					
B-natriuretic peptide BNP					
pH					
pCO_2					
pO_2					
HCO_3					

11) DIAGNOSTIC TESTS

Chest x-ray:	EKG:	Other abnormal reports:
Sputum or Blood Culture:	Other:	Other: **CAT scan**

11) MEDICATIONS   List medications and times of administration (medication administration record and check the drawer in the carts for spelling). Include over-the-counter (OTC) products/herbal medicines.

Times Due					
Brand Name		**Zofran**	**Vicodin**	**Ancef**	**Tylenol**
Generic Name	**Morphine**	**ondansetron**	**hydrocodone/ acetaminophen**	**cefazolin**	**acetaminophen**
Dose	**4 mg, every 3 hours as needed**	**4 mg, every 4 hours as needed**	**1-2 tablets every 4 to 6 hours as needed at home**	**500 mg every 4 hours for 4 doses**	**2 tablets every 4 hours as needed for temperature >101**
Administration Route	**IV**	**IV**	**po**	**IV**	**po**
Classification					
Action					
Reason This Patient is Receiving					
Pharmacokinetics	O P D 1/2 M E	O P D 1/2 M E	O P D 1/2 M E	O P D 1/2 M E	
Contraindications					
Major Adverse Side Effects					
Nursing Implications					
Pt/Family Teaching					

Developed by P. Testa, YSU

ALLERGIES/PAINS

13) Allergies: **NONE** Type of Reaction:	14) When was the last time pain medication given?
14) Where is the pain? **Abdomen**	14) How much pain is the patient in on a scale 0-10? **8/10**

TREATMENTS

15) List treatments: **Vital signs every 4 hours first 24 hours then every shift** **Pulse oximeter with vital signs, call if <92%** **Assess pain every 2 hours** **Intake and output** **Ice to incisions intermittently on and off for 15 to 20 minutes for 24 to 48 hours** **Incentive spirometer q1h while awake** **Cough & deep breath q1h while awake**
16) Support services What do support services provide for the patient?
17) What does the consultant do for the patient?:

18) DIET/FLUIDS

Type of Diet: **Clear liquids and advance as tolerated**	Restrictions:	Gag reflex intact: ☐Yes ☐No	Appetite: ☐Good ☐Fair ☐Poor	Breakfast _____ %	Lunch _____ %	Dinner _____ %
What type of diet is this?:						
What types of foods are included in this diet and what foods should be avoided?:						
Circle Those Problems That Apply:						
Prior 8 hours Fluid intake: (Oral & IV) Fluid output		• Problems: swallowing, chewing, dentures • Needs assistance with feeding • Nausea or vomiting prior to surgery • Overhydrated or dehydrated (evaluate total intake and output on flow sheet)				
Tube feedings: Type and rate		• Belching: _____ • Other: _____				

19) INTRAVENOUS FLUIDS (IV therapy record)

Type and Rate: **Lactated ringers 125/hour**	IV dressing dry, no edema, redness of site: [X] Yes [ ] No	Other:

20) ELIMINATION (flow sheet)

Last bowel movement: **Prior to admission**	Foley/condom catheter: [X] Yes [ ] No

Circle Those Problems That Apply:
• Bowel: constipation, diarrhea, flatus, incontinence, belching • Urinary: **Clear yellow urine without hesitancy, frequency, burning, incontinence, odor** • Other: _____ • What is causing the problem in elimination? _____

21) ACTIVITY (Kardex, flow sheet)

Ability to walk (gait): **Walking bent over due to pain**	Type of activity orders: **Out of bed with assistance**	Use of assistance devices: cane, walker, crutches, prosthesis:	Falls-risk assessment rating:
No. of side rails required	Restraints (flow sheet): [ ] Yes [ ] No	Weakness [X] Yes [ ] No	Trouble sleeping: [ ] Yes [ ] No

What does activity order mean?: _____ Why isn't the patient up ad lib?: _____ Would the problem cause weakness?: _____

PHYSICAL ASSESSMENT DATA

22) BP: **118/78**	2) TPR: **100.02-94-22**	23) Height: **5'10"** Weight: **145#** (nursing intake assessments)

24) NEUROLOGICAL/MENTAL STATUS:

LOC: **Alert and oriented to person, place, time** (A&O x 3), confused, etc.	Speech: **Clear, appropriate**/inappropriate
Pupils: **PERRL**	Sensory deficits for vision/hearing/taste/smell

25) MUSCULOSKELETAL STATUS:

Bones, joints, muscles (fractures, contractures, arthritis, spinal curvatures, etc):	Extremity (temperature, edema (pitting vs. nonpitting) & sensation):
Motor: **ROM x 4 extremities -Pain limits movement**	
Ted hose/plexi pulses/compression devices: type:	Casts, splint, collar, brace:

26) CARDIOVASCULAR SYSTEM:

Pulses **Radial, pedal-3+**	Capillary refill (< 3s): [X] Yes [ ] No	
Neck vein (distention):	Sounds: (S1, S2, regular) irregular: Apical rate:	Any chest pain:

27) RESPIRATORY SYSTEM:

Depth, rate, rhythm: **Non-labored**	Use of accessory muscles: **no**	Cyanosis:	Sputum color, amount:	Cough: **no**	Breath sounds: **Clear, slightly decreased in bases bilaterally**
Use of oxygen: nasal cannula, mask, tracheostomy collar:		Flow rate of oxygen:	Oxygen humidification: [ ] Yes [ ] No	Pulse oximeter: **98** % oxygen saturation	Smoking: [ ] Yes [X] No

28) GASTROINTESTINAL SYSTEM

Abdominal pain, tenderness, guarding; distension soft firm: **Slightly distended**	Bowel sounds x 4 quadrants: **Hypoactive 4 quadrants**	NG tube: describe drainage
Ostomy: describe stoma site and stools:	Other:	

29) SKIN AND WOUNDS:

Color, turgor: **Pink/elastic**	Rash, bruises:	Describe wounds (size, locations): **4 operative sites (1/2 inch each) from laparoscopy intact**	Edges approximated: [X] Yes [ ] No	Type of wound drains:
Characteristics of drainage:	Dressings: **Steri-strips clean, dry, intact**	Sutures, staples, steri-strips, other: **Steri-strips**	Risk for pressure ulcer assessment rating:	Other:

30) EYES, EARS, NOSE, THROAT (EENT):

Eyes: redness, drainage, edema, ptosis **None**	Ears: drainage **None**	Nose: redness, drainage, edema **None**	Mouth/Throat: **Pink, moist**
Psychosocial and Cultural Assessment			
31) Religious preference: **Lutheran**	32) Marital status/children/social support: **Single, mother staying with patient**	33) Health care benefits and insurance **Medical Mutual**	
34) Occupation **Student**	35) Emotional state **Anxious due to pain and unfamiliar environment, afraid to look at incisions for fear of disfigurement, cooperative, wants to go home**		

Case Study: Osteoarthritis and Dementia

1) Date of Care: **1/17/2015**	2) Patient Initials: **FS**	3) Age: **100**	3) Growth and Development **Intimacy Vs. Isolation**	4) Gender: **M**	5) Admission Date: **12/6/2010**

6) Reason for hospitalization: *Medical Dx:* **Osteoarthritis/dementia** *Pathophysiology:* **Impaired mobility, self-care deficits, and chronic confusion.**	7) Chronic illnesses: **Osteoarthritis, kyphosis, dementia, depression, benign prostatic hypertrophy, constipation, renal failure, peripheral vascular disease**
8) Name of surgical procedure: *Describe surgery:*	

9) ADVANCE DIRECTIVES (NURSE'S ADMISSION ASSESSMENTS):

Living will: [X] Yes [ ] No	Power of attorney: [X] Yes [ ] No	Do not resuscitate (DNR) order: [X] Yes [ ] No

10) LABORATORY DATA:

Test	Normal Values	Admission	Date/Time	Date/Time	Reason for Abnormal Values
White blood cells (WBCs)		10.2			
Red blood cells (RBCs)		4.04			
Hemoglobin (Hgb)		12.5			
Hematocrit (Hct)		40.3			
Platelets		323,000			
Prothrombin time (PT)					
International normalized ratio (INR)					
Activated partial thromboplastin time (Aptt)					
Sodium Na		140			
Potassium K		5.7			
Chloride Cl		108			
Glucose (FBS/BS)		90			
CO_2					
Magnesium					
Calcium					
Hemoglobin A1C					
Cholesterol					
Blood Urea Nitrogen (BUN)		21			
Creatinine		1.6			
Urine analysis (UA)		59			
Pre-albumin					
Albumin					
Calcium Ca					
Phosphate					
Bilirubin					
Alkaline phosphatase					
SGOT-Serum glutamic-oxyloacetic transaminase					
AST-Serum glutamic pyruvic transaminase					
CK					
CK MB					
Troponin					
B-natriuretic peptide BNP					
pH					
pCO_2					
pO_2					
HCO_3					

11) DIAGNOSTIC TESTS

Chest x-ray:	EKG:	Other abnormal reports:
Sputum or Blood Culture:	Other:	Other: **Recent ultrasound lower extremities—normal** **Recent urinalysis—normal**

11) MEDICATIONS   List medications and times of administration (medication administration record and check the drawer in the carts for spelling). Include over-the-counter (OTC) products/herbal medicines.

Times Due						
Brand Name	**Prozac**	**MiraLax**	**Ultram**	**Atarax**	**Tylenol**	**Dulcolax**
Generic Name	**fluoxetine**	**polyethylene glycol**	**tramadol**	**hydroxyzine**	**acetaminophen**	**biscodyl**
Dose	**10 mg, every day**	**17 grams per day (1 capful dissolved in 4 to 8 oz. liquid)**	**50 mg two times per day**	**10 mg every 6 hours as needed**	**2 tablets every 6 hours as needed**	**10 mg suppository as needed**
Administration Route	**po**	**po**	**po**	**po**	**po**	**rectal**
Classification						
Action						
Reason This Patient is Receiving						
Pharmacokinetics	O P D 1/2 M E	O P D 1/2 M E	O P D 1/2 M E	O P D 1/2 M E		
Contraindications						
Major Adverse Side Effects						
Nursing Implications						
Pt/Family Teaching						

Developed by P. Testa, YSU

ALLERGIES/PAINS

13) Allergies: **None** Type of Reaction:	14) When was the last time pain medication given?
14) Where is the pain? **Generalized**	14) How much pain is the patient in on a scale 0-10? **6/10 on rising but once up for day denies pain or discomfort**

TREATMENTS

15) List treatments:
Coat inside of nares with small amount of Vaseline every day   **Prompt voiding every 2 hours after meals**
Dycem (nonslip pad) on top of cushion in wheelchair   **Transfers with two or more hands on assist with gait belt**
Pressure reduction cushion to wheel chair   **to stand, pivot, or transfer to room**
Wheel chair or wheeled walker with staff assist   **Shower Tuesday and Friday**
Pressure reduction bed mattress   **Long sleeve shirts to protect arms**
Pacemaker check every 3 months   **Oral care for dentures and mouth care with staff assistance**
Skin check every Monday   **Active range of motion to all extremities 6 days a week**
Toileting scheduling on rising, before and after immediately   **Alcohol drink per request (drinks beer in evening)**
**   after meals**

16) Support services What do support services provide for the patient?

17) What does the consultant do for the patient?:

18) DIET/FLUIDS

Type of Diet: **Regular, soft foods, prune juice daily for breakfast**	Restrictions: **No added salt**	Gag reflex intact: [X] Yes [ ] No	Appetite: [X] Good [ ] Fair [ ] Poor	Breakfast **90** %	Lunch **90** %	Dinner **90** %

What type of diet is this?:
What types of foods are included in this diet and what foods should be avoided?:

Circle Those Problems That Apply:	
Prior 8 hours Fluid intake: (Oral & IV) Fluid output Tube feedings: Type and rate	• Needs assistance with feeding • Nausea or vomiting prior to surgery • Overhydrated or dehydrated (evaluate total intake and output on flow sheet) • Belching: _____ • Other: _____

19) INTRAVENOUS FLUIDS (IV therapy record)

Type and Rate:	IV dressing dry, no edema, redness of site: ☐ Yes ☐ No	Other:

20) ELIMINATION (flow sheet)

Last bowel movement: **Daily**	Foley/condom catheter: ☐ Yes ☒ No

Circle Those Problems That Apply:

- Bowel: constipation, diarrhea, flatus, incontinence, belching
- Urinary: **Clear yellow urine without hesitancy, frequency, burning, incontinence, odor**
- Other: _____
- What is causing the problem in elimination? _____

21) ACTIVITY

Ability to walk (gait): **Unsteady—can only walk a few steps, wheel chair dependent for mobility**	Type of activity orders: **2 assistants for movement**	Use of assistance devices: cane, walker, crutches, prosthesis: **Gait belt, wheel chair**	Falls-risk: **High**
No. of side rails required	Restraints (flow sheet): ☐ Yes ☒ No	Weakness ☒ Yes ☐ No	Trouble sleeping: ☐ Yes ☐ No

What does activity order mean?: _____
Why isn't the patient up ad lib?: _____
Would the problem cause weakness?: _____

PHYSICAL ASSESSMENT DATA

22) BP: **142/72**	2) TPR: **97.3-72-18**	23) Height: **5'5"** Weight: **130#** (nursing intake assessments)

24) NEUROLOGICAL/MENTAL STATUS:

LOC: **Alert and oriented to person often becomes confused about place, time and situation**	Speech: **Clear, at times inappropriate**
Pupils: **PERRL**	Sensory deficits for **vision—Glasses**/hearing/taste/smell

25) MUSCULOSKELETAL STATUS:

Bones, joints, muscles: **Osteoarthritis and kyphosis**	Extremity: **Weakness of legs, no edema, cool lower extremities**
Motor: **ROM decreased in all extremities**	
Ted hose/plexi pulses/compression devices: type:	Casts, splint, collar, brace:

26) CARDIOVASCULAR SYSTEM:

Pulses (Radial), (pedal) palpable	Capillary refill (< 3s): ☒ Yes ☐ No
Neck vein (distention):	Sounds: (S1, S2, regular) irregular: Apical rate:	Any chest pain: **None**

27) RESPIRATORY SYSTEM:

Depth, rate, rhythm: **Non-labored**	Use of accessory muscles: **No**	Cyanosis:	Sputum color, amount:	Cough: **No**	Breath sounds: **Clear**
Use of oxygen: nasal cannula, mask, tracheostomy collar:	Flow rate of oxygen:	Oxygen humidification: ☐ Yes ☐ No	Pulse oximeter: **98** % oxygen saturation		Smoking: ☐ Yes ☒ No

28) GASTROINTESTINAL SYSTEM

Abdominal pain, tenderness, guarding; distension soft firm: **Soft non-distended**	Bowel sounds x 4 quadrants: **Present**	NG tube: describe drainage
Ostomy: describe stoma site and stools:	Other:	

29) SKIN AND WOUNDS:

Color, turgor: **Pink/decreased elasticity**	Rash, bruises: **None**	Describe wounds (size, locations): **None**	Edges approximated: ☐ Yes ☐ No	Type of wound drains:
Characteristics of drainage:	Dressings:	Sutures, staples, steri-strips, other:	Risk for pressure ulcer assessment rating: **High**	Other: **Thin "tissue paper" skin over hands, arms, lower legs and feet**

30) EYES, EARS, NOSE, THROAT (EENT):

Eyes: redness, drainage, edema, ptosis **None**	Ears: drainage **None**	Nose: redness, drainage, edema **Pink, moist**	Mouth/Throat: **Pink, moist**
Psychosocial and Cultural Assessment			
31) Religious preference: **Catholic**	32) Marital status/children/social support: **Widowed, family has fixed room with pictures of the past to help keep him oriented. Family supportive but do not visit frequently because they live in different parts of the state. Participates in group activities such as church, bingo, listening to music.**		33) Health care benefits and insurance: **Medicare**
34) Occupation **Retired physician**	35) Emotional state **Anxious and becomes frustrated and pounds on table when he forgets what he was going to do next, he was very intelligent and now he can't remember basic things.**		

Index

Note: Page numbers followed by a "b" indicated boxed material, page numbers followed by "f" indicate figures, and page numbers followed by "t" indicate tables.